TODDLERS MOVING & LEARNING

Other Redleaf Press Books by Rae Pica

Preschoolers & Kindergartners Moving & Learning

Early Elementary Children Moving & Learning

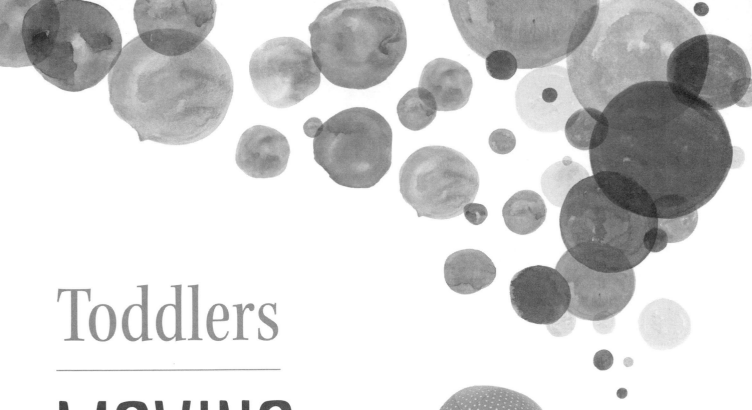

Toddlers

MOVING & LEARNING

RAE PICA

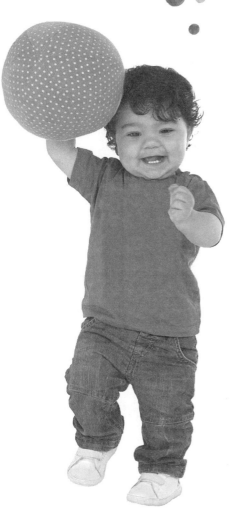

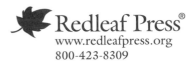 **Redleaf Press**®
www.redleafpress.org
800-423-8309

Published by Redleaf Press
10 Yorkton Court
St. Paul, MN 55117
www.redleafpress.org

First edition 2014
Cover design by Ryan Scheife, Mayfly Design
Cover artwork composed from images: (empty room) ssstep/iStockphoto; (watercolor circles abstract and colored spots) crisserbug/iStockphoto; (toddler with a ball) alexandrenunes/Veer
Interior design by Ryan Scheife, Mayfly Design
Typeset in Kepler MM
Interior illustrations by Chris Wold Dyrud
Printed in the United States of America
21 20 19 18 17 16 15 14   1 2 3 4 5 6 7 8

Guidelines on pages 10–11 are from *Active Start: A Statement of Physical Activity Guidelines for Children from Birth to Age 5*, 2nd ed., by the American Alliance for Health, Physical Education, Recreation and Dance (AAHPERD) (Reston, VA: AAHPERD, 2009). Reprinted with permission.

Excerpts on page 12 are from *Developmentally Appropriate Practice in Early Childhood Programs Serving Children from Birth through Age 8*, a position statement by National Association for the Education of Young Children (NAEYC). Copyright © 2009 NAEYC. www.naeyc.org/files/naeyc/file/positions/PSDAP.pdf. Reprinted with permission.

Excerpts on pages 11–12 are from *NAEYC Standards for Early Childhood Professional Preparation Programs*, a position statement by NAEYC. Copyright © 2009 NAEYC. http://www.naeyc.org/files/naeyc/file/positions/ProfPrepStandards09.pdf. Reprinted with permission.

Library of Congress Cataloging-in-Publication Data
Pica, Rae, 1953-
  Toddlers moving and learning / Rae Pica.
      pages cm
  Summary: "Movement activities can help toddlers channel their energy in creative and beneficial ways as they learn healthy habits. This physical education curriculum includes a variety of lesson plans and activities that support toddlers' movement in developmentally appropriate ways" — Provided by publisher.
  Includes bibliographical references.
  ISBN 978-1-60554-267-6
  1. Toddlers—Development. 2. Physical education for children.   I. Title.
  HQ774.5.P53 2014
  612.6'54—dc23
                                  2013031259

Printed on acid-free paper

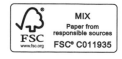

The three books in the Moving & Learning series
are dedicated to my "angel," Fredrick Davis.
He knows why.

Contents

Acknowledgments

I couldn't be happier that the Moving & Learning series is finding a home at Redleaf Press. It's become clear to me that this is where these books belong. I'd like to thank Kyra Ostendorf and David Heath for the warm welcome, with extra-special thanks to David for being a fabulous editor. Working with you was such a pleasure!

I'm forever grateful to Richard Gardzina for the original music that accompanies these curriculum packages. He is a remarkable composer, and what I especially love about what he created here is that he never considered it "children's" music. Instead, he set out to compose and perform the best music he could.

Special thanks to the children and teachers with whom I've worked over the years—those on whom I "practiced" and those who've embraced the "movement message" at my presentations. Your enthusiasm, along with your expressions of appreciation over the years, has kept me going!

Deep appreciation to my mom, whose pride in me warms my heart.

Activity Chart

Lesson	Body-Parts Activities	Nonlocomotor Activities	Locomotor Activities	Movement-Element Activities
1	Heads, Bellies, Toes	Let's Stretch	Let's Walk	Exploring Up and Down
2	Show Me	Let's Bend	Let's Run	Exploring Straight and Round
3	Flexing/Pointing Feet	Let's Shake	Let's Jump	Shapes in Motion
4	Where Is Thumbkin?	Let's Sway	Tiny Steps/Giant Steps	Up and Down Make-Believe
5	Open and Close	Let's Turn	Let's Gallop	Pop Goes the Weasel
6	The Wash Song	Bending and Stretching	Let's Creep	Moving Slow/Moving Fast
7	See My Hands	Let's Strike	Let's Roll	The Bumblebee
8	See My Feet	Let's Push and Pull	Marching Band	Moving Backward
9	See My Face	The Tightrope	Follow the Leader	Marching Slow/Marching Fast
10	Mirror Game	Let's Lift	Moving Like the Animals	Slow-Motion Moving
11	Simon Says	Let's Balance	Let's Tiptoe	The Tiptoe Song
12	The Body Song	Shake, Wiggle, and Vibrate	Let's Jump Again	Moving Softly/Moving Loudly
13	Body-Part Balance	High and Low	Let's Crawl	Robots and Astronauts
14	Traveling Body Parts	In My Space	Follow the Leader	Common Meters

Curriculum Connectors Chart

Lesson	Activity	Art	Language Arts	Math	Music	Science	Social Studies	Page
1	Heads, Bellies, Toes		X		X	X		28
1	Let's Stretch	X	X	X		X		29
1	Let's Walk		X		X		X	31
1	Exploring Up and Down	X		X				33
2	Show Me					X		36
2	Let's Bend			X		X		37
2	Let's Run		X		X			38
2	Exploring Straight and Round	X		X			X	39
3	Flexing/Pointing Feet		X					42
3	Let's Shake		X		X			44
3	Let's Jump			X	X	X		45
3	Shapes in Motion	X	X	X				47
4	Where Is Thumbkin?		X	X	X			50
4	Let's Sway				X	X		51
4	Tiny Steps/Giant Steps	X	X	X				52
4	Up and Down Make-Believe			X		X		53
5	Open and Close		X		X	X		56
5	Let's Turn		X		X			57
5	Let's Gallop		X		X	X		59
5	Pop Goes the Weasel		X	X	X			60
6	The Wash Song		X		X	X		62
6	Bending and Stretching	X		X				64
6	Let's Creep		X			X		65
6	Moving Slow/Moving Fast			X	X	X	X	66
7	See My Hands		X		X	X		70
7	Let's Strike		X		X		X	72
7	Let's Roll		X		X			74
7	The Bumblebee		X		X	X		75
8	See My Feet					X		78
8	Let's Push and Pull					X		79
8	Marching Band				X		X	81
8	Moving Backward	X	X	X				83
9	See My Face		X			X	X	86
9	The Tightrope				X	X	X	88
9	Follow the Leader	X	X		X			90

(CONTINUED ON NEXT PAGE)

Curriculum Connectors Chart (continued)

Lesson	Activity	Art	Language Arts	Math	Music	Science	Social Studies	Page
9	Marching Slow/Marching Fast			X	X		X	91
10	Mirror Game	X	X			X		94
10	Let's Lift			X		X		95
10	Moving Like the Animals					X		97
10	Slow-Motion Moving			X	X			98
11	Simon Says		X		X	X		100
11	Let's Balance	X		X		X		102
11	Let's Tiptoe					X		104
11	The Tiptoe Song		X	X	X			105
12	The Body Song	X	X	X	X	X		108
12	Shake, Wiggle, and Vibrate					X		109
12	Let's Jump Again	X		X				110
12	Moving Softly/Moving Loudly				X	X		111
13	Body-Part Balance			X		X		114
13	High and Low	X	X	X	X			115
13	Let's Crawl		X			X		117
13	Robots and Astronauts				X	X	X	118
14	Traveling Body Parts	X		X		X		120
14	In My Space	X	X	X	X			121
14	Follow the Leader	X	X	X		X		122
14	Common Meters			X	X			123

Song List

Title	Length	Page
"Walking Along"	1:51	31
"The Track Meet"	1:04	38
"Wiggle, Wiggle, Shake and Giggle"	1:22	44
"Rabbits and 'Roos"	1:02	45
"Where Is Thumbkin?"	2:07	50
"The Swaying Song"	1:27	51
"Open and Close"	1:34	56
"Pop Goes the Weasel"	1:10	60
"The Wash Song"	1:42	62
"Moving Slow/Moving Fast"	1:26	66
"Hands-Hands-Hands"	1:48	70
"The Bumblebee"	1:07	75
"Marching Band"	1:46	81
"Circus Medley"	3:55	88
"Marching Slow/Marching Fast"	1:31	91
"Slow-Motion Moving"	1:21	98
"The Tiptoe Song"	1:04	105
"The Body Song"	2:11	108
"Moving Softly/Moving Loudly"	1:30	111
"High and Low"	1:13	115
"Robots and Astronauts"	1:46	118
"In My Space"	2:42	121
"Common Meters"	2:14	123

Introduction

Toddlers, perhaps even more than older children, need to move—to channel their energies in creative, beneficial ways and get started on the right foot, as it were, toward proper development. So, not surprisingly, teachers and caregivers who knew of my materials for preschoolers began asking for movement activities and music they could use successfully with toddlers.

Of course, "watering down" my preschool program wasn't an option. In fact, because there are so many differences between toddlers (for this book, considered to be children ages eighteen to thirty-six months old) and children just two years older, there was little of *Preschoolers & Kindergartners* that would be usable. Songs had to be shortened and, in many cases, slowed down. And naturally, new songs and activities had to be written.

The result is the movement program in your hands—*Toddlers*—which is now being used in schools, child care settings, recreation centers, and gyms throughout the United States and in several other countries.

The curriculum consists of fourteen lesson plans with four activities per plan (not including extensions). Each lesson is intended to take approximately thirty minutes to complete. (Alternatives are discussed later, under "Implementing the Program.") The fourteen lessons and their activities have been arranged in a developmental progression, from least to most challenging, with each lesson plan consisting of one body-parts activity, one nonlocomotor activity, one locomotor skill experience, and one activity exploring an element of movement.

The lessons begin with simple body-part identification, which is the basis of any movement program. The lessons also start with the simplest locomotor skills (movements that transport the body from one place to another) of walking and running. (Technically, crawling and creeping are the simplest, but the exploration of these skills has been placed later in order to promote a sense of "maturity" among the children.) The simplest nonlocomotor skills (movements performed while remaining in one place) of bending and stretching are also found in early lessons, along with the simplest movement elements of space and shape.

I believe very much in the importance of beginning at the beginning and progressing in a logical, developmental manner. Not only can we expect greater success from children who are encouraged to build upon their earlier successes as stepping stones, but we can expect greater *response* from them as well. Early in my own teaching experiences, I was guilty of asking children to respond to challenges with which they could not possibly be comfortable; they hadn't progressed through the stages necessary to *make* them comfortable. The result was intimidation and a lot of blank stares—and no wonder. It was similar to asking a fledgling ballet student to perform a perfectly executed *tour en l'air* (turn in the air) without first acquainting her or him with the basic balletic skills!

The idea is to make the children feel good about experiencing movement by starting slowly and providing them with frequent opportunities to experience success.

Because children need opportunities to explore movement on its own, to find and use their own personal rhythms, not all of the activities in this book are accompanied by music. (Activities using music have been marked with a musical note: ♪.) However, children do love music—and it does contribute much to movement experiences—so I have included it wherever it could make a contribution to the learning experience. The songs that are part of this program are almost entirely original, having been written specifically for the activities they accompany. They make it possible for teachers to add the joy and energy of music to movement experiences without the effort of having to first *locate* appropriate music, and they make it possible for the children to better understand such abstract concepts as slow and fast, light and heavy, and bound and free. The songs expose the children to both electronic and acoustic instruments and to as many musical elements as I could manage to include. I believe in variety, and variety is what this curriculum offers the children, and you!

Finally, every activity in *Toddlers* includes some simple questions to help you evaluate whether or not the children are meeting the activity's objectives and Curriculum Connectors, pointing out ways in which the activity correlates, or can be made to correlate, with other content areas. Also, while it is my feeling that the body is the most important piece of equipment in movement experiences, I realize that using actual equipment can add another dimension to—and increase the challenge of—an activity. So, where appropriate, the section Adding Equipment has been included, offering suggestions for the use of hoops, scarves, streamers, and other props generally available in early childhood classrooms.

Benefits of Moving & Learning

Movement experiences in general—and this curriculum specifically—have many benefits for children. They exercise the whole body, including the mind, and not just the muscles; they create a love of movement that should develop into a lifetime desire for physical fitness; and their success-oriented philosophy provides numerous opportunities for learning, participating, and enjoying. The following are some of their more specific benefits.

Physical Development

Perhaps the simplest and most important reason children should be allowed and encouraged to move is to develop movement skills.

Although it is commonly believed children automatically acquire motor skills as their bodies develop, maturation only means that children will be able to execute most movement skills at a low performance level. Continuous practice and instruction are needed if the child's performance level and movement repertoire are to increase (Gallahue and Cleland Donnelly 2003). In other words, once a child is able to creep and walk, gross-motor skills should be taught—just as other abilities are taught. Furthermore, special attention should be paid to children demonstrating gross-motor delays, as such delays will not simply disappear over time.

As Linda Carson explains, families and teachers "would not advocate learning to read or communicate by having their children enter a 'gross cognitive area' where children could engage in self-selected 'reading play' with a variety of books" (2001, 9). Similarly, engaging in unplanned, self-selected physical activities—or even a movement learning center—is not enough for young children to gain movement skills.

Why does the development of motor skills matter, when not every child will go on to become an athlete or a dancer? It matters because children who feel confident in their movement skills are likely to continue moving throughout their lives. And that's significant because of the many health problems that can be attributed to sedentary living.

Although children love to move—and adults tend to think of them as constantly being in motion—children today are leading much more sedentary lives than did their predecessors. According to Nielsen research, "Younger children age 2–5 log close to 25 hours of TV time each week, more than 4.5 hours watching their favorite DVDs, about 1.5 hours viewing DVR offerings, more than an hour competing at video games and 45 minutes with the VCR" (McDonough 2009). In fact, watching television is the predominant sedentary behavior in children, second only to sleeping (Kaur et al. 2003). The advent of computers and video games has also contributed to the decline in activity. A study from the Kaiser Family Foundation determined that children ages eight to eighteen are spending more than seven and a half hours a day with electronic devices (Lewin 2010)—the same number of hours some people spend at full-time jobs.

According to Bar-Or et al., there is one consistent observation that stands out among the studies of energy expenditures in young children: children under the age of seven seem to expend about 20 to 30 percent less energy in physical activity than the level recommended by the World Health Organization (1998). The Children's Activity and Movement in Preschools Study (CHAMPS) determined that children enrolled in preschools were "engaged in moderate to vigorous physical activity (MVPA) during only 3.4 percent of the preschool day" (NIEER 2010, 12). Pate et al. observed two thousand children and found that "children attending preschools were engaged in MVPA during only 2.6% of observation intervals. During over 85% of intervals, children were engaged in either very light activity or sedentary behaviors" (2008, 443).

Considered together, these factors provide cause for concern regarding children's fitness levels. Statistics indicate that 40 percent of five- to eight-year-olds show at least one heart disease risk factor, including hypertension and obesity. The latter, which is on the rise, particularly among children, has been linked to television viewing (Bar-Or et al. 1998). A Canadian study determined that the blood vessels of obese children have a stiffness normally seen in much older adults who have cardiovascular disease (Science Daily 2010). Furthermore, the Centers for Disease Control and Prevention (CDC) estimates that American children born in the year 2000 face a one-in-three chance of developing type 2 diabetes, previously known as adult-onset diabetes because it was rarely seen in children (2008).

A developmentally appropriate movement curriculum, such as *Toddlers*, can give children the practice and instruction necessary to refine their movement skills and expand their movement vocabularies. Moreover, with *Toddlers*, children have the opportunity to frequently experience success, which makes movement pleasurable for them. Thus they are more likely to become (and stay!) physically fit.

Social/Emotional Development

Marianne Frostig, in her classic book *Movement Education: Theory and Practice*, states,

> Movement education can help a child to adjust socially and emotionally because it can provide him with successful experiences and permit interrelationships with other children in groups and with a partner. Movement education requires that a child be aware of others in [activities] in which he shares space . . . ; he has to take turns and to cooperate. He thus develops social awareness and achieves satisfaction through peer relationships and group play. (1970, 26)

This program provides opportunities for successful experiences, and it permits interrelationships with other children. Even before the children are asked to work cooperatively with partners and groups, they must be aware of others around them, adjusting their movement patterns to avoid collisions.

This book also offers a blend of teacher-directed activities and a creative problem-solving approach to instruction. The latter lends itself to success by allowing children to respond to challenges at their own developmental levels and rates. This approach increases children's self-confidence (and thus their self-esteem) as they see their choices being accepted and praised. According to Muska Mosston and Sara Ashworth, two important results of problem solving are the "development of patience with peers and the enhancement of respect for other people's ideas" (1990, 259).

The development of *empathy* is also promoted through exposure to certain social issues that will hopefully make positive impressions in your toddlers' young and open minds. For example, to physically imitate the movements and characteristics of a variety of animals is to imagine what it is like to *be* those animals. Those of us who wish to see children raised with a healthy respect and compassion for the world's creatures can certainly hope that, once our children have imagined what it's like to be the animals, they will never be able to imagine a world *without* them.

Cognitive Development

It has been said that joy is the most powerful of all mental stimuli. For young children, movement is certainly joyous. Beyond that, however, studies of how young children learn have proven that they especially acquire knowledge experientially—through play, experimentation, exploration, and discovery.

For example, when children move over, under, around, through, beside, and near objects and others, they better grasp the meaning of these prepositions and geometry concepts. When they perform a "slow walk" or skip "lightly," adjectives and adverbs become much more than abstract ideas. When they're given the opportunity to physically demonstrate such action words as *stomp*, *pounce*, *stalk*, or *slither*—or descriptive words such as *smooth*, *strong*, *gentle*, or *enormous*—word comprehension is immediate and long lasting. The words are *in context*, as opposed to being a mere collection of letters. This is what promotes emergent literacy and a love of language.

Similarly, if children take on high, low, wide, and narrow body shapes, they'll have a much greater understanding of these quantitative concepts—and opposites—than do children who are merely presented with the words and their definitions. When they act out the lyrics to "Ten in the Bed" ("There were five in the bed, and the little one said, 'Roll over' . . ."), they can *see* that five minus one leaves four. The same understanding—and fascination—results when children have personal experience with such scientific concepts as gravity, flotation, evaporation, magnetics, balance and stability, and action and reaction.

Additionally, learning by doing creates more neural networks in the brain and throughout the body, making the entire body a tool for learning (Hannaford 2005).

There is a growing body of research determining that physical activity activates the brain much more so than doing seatwork. While sitting increases fatigue and reduces concentration, moderate- to vigorous-intensity movement feeds oxygen, water, and glucose to the brain, optimizing its performance.

Beyond providing an opportunity for children to "feed" their brain and to learn by doing, *Toddlers* contributes to cognitive development in the following ways:

- These movement experiences offer numerous opportunities for the children to deal with the concepts of space and shape. Thus they will be learning to deal with abstract thought. Since language, numbers, and the alphabet are all abstractions, this is very necessary preparation.
- The children will have considerable opportunities to experience directionality and spatial awareness, which are critical to reading and writing abilities.
- By using a problem-solving method of instruction with the children, you will be enhancing their problem-solving capabilities. They are going to discover there will always be more than one way to solve any problem or to meet any challenge.
- The children will experience cross-lateral movement, which helps children cross the body's midline and activates both hemispheres of the brain in a balanced way. Because such movements involve both of the eyes, ears, hands, and feet, as well as core muscles on both sides of the body, they activate both hemispheres and all four lobes of the brain. This means cognitive functioning is heightened and learning becomes easier (Hannaford 2005).
- Body image influences a child's emotional health, learning ability, and intellectual performance.

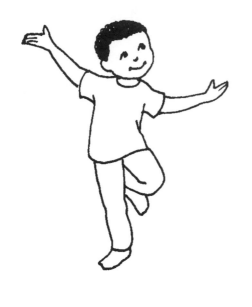
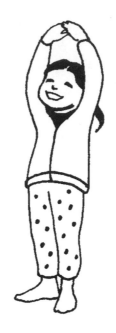
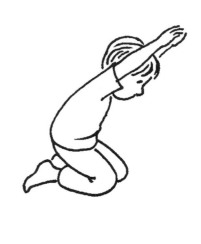

Creative Development

Can you imagine a world without creativity and self-expression—not just in the arts, but in science, business and industry, education, and life itself?

Can you honestly say you do not find some creativity in each toddler you work with—or that you do not know at least one adult who has lost the ability to express himself or herself creatively or otherwise? Where does creativity go from the time we are toddlers to the time we become adults? Is that loss of potential a result of a society and an educational system that fail to emphasize creativity and individuality?

Why is creativity important? There are a lot of reasons. However, for young children, creativity means there is no one *right* answer. This enhances their sense of mastery, which in turn promotes their self-esteem and helps them realize they can indeed have some effect on their environment.

Teresa M. Amabile reported that the key personality traits of highly creative people, if not naturally occurring, can be developed in childhood. These traits include

- self-discipline about work;
- perseverance even when frustrated;
- independence;
- tolerance for unclear situations;

- nonconformity to society's stereotypes;
- ability to wait for rewards;
- self-motivation to do excellent work; and
- a willingness to take risks.
  (1992)

According to Mary Mayesky,

> Adults who work with young children are in an especially crucial position to foster each child's creativity. In the day-to-day experiences in early childhood settings, as young children actively explore their world, adults' attitudes clearly transmit their feelings to the child. A child who meets with unquestionable acceptance of her unique approach to the world will feel safe in expressing her creativity, whatever the activity or situation. (2009, 24)

Toddlers encourages children to find their *own* ways of responding to challenges, to be individuals, and to *imagine*. When you meet their uniqueness with "unquestionable acceptance," the children will be better equipped later in their lives to imagine solutions to problems they face, to feel empathy, and to plan futures that are full and satisfying.

As Margaret Newell H'Doubler so aptly writes in her classic book, *The Dance and Its Place in Education,*

> as every child has a right to a box of crayons and certain instruction in the fundamental principles of the art of drawing, whether there is any chance of his ever becoming a great artist or not, so every child has a right to know how to obtain control of his body so that he may use it, to the limit of his abilities, for the expression of his reactions to life. (1925, 33)

Benefits to Children with Special Needs

All of the benefits previously cited can be applied to children with special needs. Additionally, coordination, listening skills, conceptual learning, and expressive ability are just a few of the areas enhanced through regular participation—at whatever level possible—in movement experiences.

Perhaps of greatest importance, however, is the contribution that movement experiences can make toward the special child's self-concept. Often children with disabilities fail to form a complete body image due to exclusion from physical activity. Similarly, because they do not necessarily perform the same way other children do, they develop a distorted body image (Gallahue and Cleland Donnelly 2003). Identifying and moving various body parts can "help the child discover how each body part fits into the whole schema of a human body. This enables the child to explore body boundaries and define his/her body image" (Samuelson 1981, 53). Achieving regular success in movement activities will contribute greatly to the child's confidence—perhaps offering for the first time an opportunity to feel good about himself or herself.

Another unique opportunity derived from the movement program is the chance to be part of a group. As the child's self-concept becomes more developed, he is better able to relate to others. As the child's movements and ideas are regularly accepted and valued, he receives greater acceptance from his peers. Becoming part of a group—making contributions, taking turns, following rules—has the additional benefit of enhancing social skills.

Meeting Standards

In today's educational climate, meeting standards is a consideration for all education professionals, including those in early childhood. Movement experiences in general, and those in *Toddlers* specifically, can address multiple standards outlined by the American Alliance for Health, Physical Education, Recreation and Dance (AAHPERD) and the National Association for the Education of Young Children (NAEYC).

For example, the position of AAHPERD in *Active Start: A Statement of Physical Activity Guidelines for Children from Birth to Age 5* is that "all children from birth to age 5 should engage daily in physical activity that promotes movement skillfulness and foundations of health-related fitness" (AAHPERD 2009, iv). For toddlers specifically, their guidelines include the following:

1. Toddlers should engage in a total of at least 30 minutes of structured physical activity each day.

2. Toddlers should engage in at least 60 minutes—and up to several hours—per day of unstructured physical activity and should not be sedentary for more than 60 minutes at a time, except when sleeping.

3. Toddlers should be given ample opportunities to develop movement skills that will serve as the building blocks for future motor skillfulness and physical activity.

4. Toddlers should have access to indoor and outdoor areas that meet or exceed recommended safety standards for performing large-muscle activities.

5. Those in charge of toddlers' well-being are responsible for understanding the importance of physical activity and promoting movement skills by providing opportunities for structured and unstructured physical activity and movement experiences. (AAHPERD 2009, 7, 8, 9, 10, and 11)

NAEYC offers *Standards for Early Childhood Professional Preparation Programs*. Among those standards addressed by *Toddlers* are the following:

- Standard 1a: Knowing and understanding young children's characteristics and needs.
- Standard 1b: Knowing and understanding the multiple influences on development and learning.
- Standard 1c: Using developmental knowledge to create healthy, respectful, supportive, and challenging learning environments.
- Standard 3b: Knowing about and using observation, documentation, and other appropriate assessment tools and approaches.
- Standard 4a: Understanding positive relationships and supportive interactions as the foundation of their work with children.
- Standard 4b: Knowing and understanding effective strategies and tools for early education.
- Standard 4c: Using a broad repertoire of developmentally appropriate teaching/learning approaches.
- Standard 5a: Understanding content knowledge and resources in academic disciplines.

- Standard 5b: Knowing and using the central concepts, inquiry tools, and structures of content areas or academic disciplines.
- Standard 5c: Using their own knowledge, appropriate early learning standards, and other resources to design, implement, and evaluate meaningful, challenging curricula for each child.
  (2009b, 11, 13, 14, and 16)

NAEYC's position statement *Developmentally Appropriate Practice in Early Childhood Programs Serving Children from Birth through Age 8* specifies that "all the domains of development and learning—physical, social and emotional, and cognitive—are important, and they are closely interrelated. Children's development and learning in one domain influence and are influenced by what takes place in other domains" (2009a, 11). The position statement instructs teachers to "plan curriculum experiences that integrate children's learning *within* and *across* the domains (physical, social, emotional, cognitive) and the disciplines (including language, literacy, mathematics, social studies, science, art, music, physical education, and health)" (2009a, 21).

Implementing the Program

In truth, the term *lesson plan*, as it is used in this program, is not technically correct, but I have used it because a suitable substitute does not seem to exist. Typically, a lesson plan specifies details for teaching *one class period* of a learning unit. But it was my intention that teachers using this book would be able to create as many lessons as they wanted—or deemed necessary—from each of my plans. Because I purposely built a great deal of flexibility into the book, there are probably as many ways to use these lesson plans as there are teachers!

In other words, the fact that there are four activities per plan does not mean that you must complete all four every time you schedule a movement session. Similarly, you should not feel as though you have to use the lesson plans exactly as they are laid out. Although I certainly hope you will keep the developmental progression of the activities and their extensions in mind as you go through them, I realize that nobody knows your toddlers better than you do. So you should not hesitate to adapt the lesson plans, perhaps abbreviating activities or changing their order, if you feel it is better for your children. If certain activities are too advanced for your toddlers, feel free to pass them by and return to them later; they are offered here simply as possibilities.

You may decide, for instance, that you wish to explore one activity and all of its extensions in a series of movement sessions before moving on to the next activity on the page. Or you might choose to ignore the extensions until you have run through all fourteen lesson plans, at which time you return to Lesson 1 and begin again with the first suggested extension under each activity.

Another option is to add a specific warm-up exercise (a favorite finger-play or song, perhaps) to the beginning of each lesson. Performing the same warm-up all the time can serve to alert your children to the fact that it is movement time. You can finish with a cooldown of your choice too. For instance, pretending to melt puts closure on the day's lesson by offering children a chance to relax and to lower themselves to the floor, where they can await information about what comes next.

The one suggestion I would strongly recommend is that you implement lots of repetition. As an early childhood professional, you recognize how important repetition is to young children—especially toddlers. Just because a movement activity appears only once in these lesson plans doesn't mean it is intended to be experienced only once! You should repeat activities and even whole lessons as often as necessary to ensure success.

Will you do movement only as part of circle time, or will you schedule longer movement sessions? Will you schedule sessions weekly, daily, or something in between? The following section of the introduction attempts to help you answer some of those questions and provides information you will need to make the best possible use of this book.

Scheduling Movement Experiences

As mentioned earlier, each of the lesson plans in this program consists of four activities and is intended to take approximately thirty minutes to complete. Whether that holds true for you depends largely upon your particular situation. Some groups of toddlers are not ready to sustain interest in anything for thirty minutes, while others are delighted to "play" with you for half an hour. If you have a very small group of children, or if you have had to divide a large group in half because of lack of space, you may find that you are able to move through a lesson plan more quickly. If you have more eighteen-month-olds in your class than three-year-olds, you may find that it takes the younger ones longer to complete a single lesson—or that you cannot keep their attention long enough to complete all four activities. Because of the nature of children in general, it is even possible that one lesson will last thirty minutes, the next only twenty minutes, and the following just fifteen!

In other words, you will have to be prepared to play it by ear. However, that should not be a problem. If you have not completed a lesson when your time is up, you can simply pick up where you left off next time. If your class runs short, you can always repeat activities from previous lessons.

My hope, of course, is that you will plan for a daily movement session. If you do movement on a daily basis, I suggest using no more than two *Moving & Learning* lesson plans per week, repeating the activities in those two lessons throughout the week. Otherwise, the children's senses will be overloaded and focusing will be much more difficult.

Finally, should you wish to adapt the lesson plans, remember that a lesson should include both large and small movements whenever possible. In most cases, this also means that the lesson will consist of both vigorous and not-so-vigorous activities—which you will definitely want to alternate, for your sake as well as the children's.

Creating a Positive Learning Environment

Success is always the goal in a *Moving & Learning* program, so the atmosphere of your class plays an important role. Classroom management must be handled with special care. With so much activity involved, however, maintaining control is not always easy.

But children love to move—and they like to show off and display their abilities—especially to you. You can use this to your advantage when presenting challenges. If you introduce the challenges with a phrase like "Show me you can" or "Let me see you," the children will want to show you they can. It is a simple technique, but amazingly effective!

There are fewer behavioral problems when a program is success oriented from the beginning. A child who is experiencing success is less likely to become bored or want to disrupt the class.

There are, however, two important rules you should explain to the children in the beginning and enforce consistently. The first is that there are to be *no collisions*. In fact, there should be no touching unless it happens to be a specific part of an activity. To phrase this positively, you can say, "We will give each other enough space to move" or "We will always leave enough space for our friends." At the start this may be difficult to enforce, especially with the youngest children—because they generally enjoy colliding with one another! So it is your challenge to make it a goal for the children *not* to interfere with one another.

You can accomplish this by asking the children to space themselves evenly at the beginning of every movement session (carpet squares or hoops can help with this). Explain the idea of personal space to them, perhaps by encouraging the children to imagine they are each surrounded by a giant bubble; whether standing still or moving, they should avoid causing any of the bubbles to burst. Another image that works quite successfully is that of dolphins swimming. Children who have seen these creatures in action, either at an aquarium or on television, will be able to relate to the fact that dolphins swim side by side but never get close enough to touch one another. The goal, then, is for the children to behave similarly. (Providing pictures of dolphins swimming together would also be helpful.)

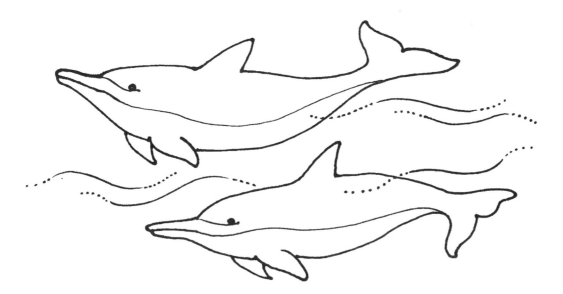

The second rule that will contribute to a manageable and pleasant environment is that there can be *no noise* (which differs from *no sound*), ensuring that your challenges, directions, and follow-up questions can be heard at all times, with no need for shouting. To phrase this positively, explain that the children are to move as *quietly* as possible. You can accomplish this by establishing a signal that indicates it is time to stop, look, and listen: "Stop, look at me, and listen for what comes next." Choose a signal the children should *watch* for, like two fingers held in the air or the appearance of a special prop (for example, a puppet or a scarf) or something they must *listen* for—like a hand clap, a strike on a triangle, or three taps on a drum—and make it their "secret code." A whistle is generally not suitable, as it can be heard above a great deal of noise, which means the children will know they can create a ruckus and still hear your signal. (In the same way that a whisper is more effective than a shout, you want a quieter signal that the children have to be *listening* for.) Nor will your voice be effective, as it is heard so often by the children.

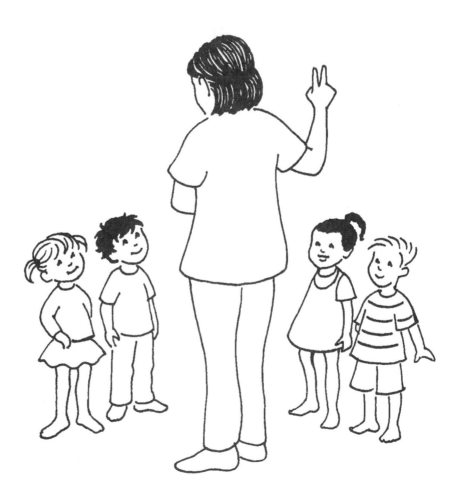

If a child acts out, distracting other children, ask the child to sit on the sidelines and act as an audience member. Give him or her the responsibility of deciding when to rejoin the activities by stating, "When you're ready to join us again, let me know." Whether the child is on the sidelines by request or is simply reluctant to participate, she or he should be allowed to observe only.

In general, as in all matters relating to movement education, a positive attitude is the key. Movement activities should take place in a friendly, encouraging, and fun atmosphere, balanced with some basic ground rules for human behavior. This atmosphere, together with the fact that the children are experiencing success, will ensure that behavioral problems will be minimal.

Suggested Attire

Whenever possible, the children should move in unrestrictive clothing—for obvious reasons. The most important contribution to effective movement is probably the *bare foot*.

Children have worn sneakers during physical activity for so long now that we seem to have forgotten that the feet do have sentient qualities. They can grip the floor for strength and balance, and the foot consists of different parts (toes, ball, heel) that can be more easily felt and used when bare. Besides, young children feel a natural affinity for the ground, which can be enhanced by stripping away all the barriers between it and the feet.

Of course, sometimes it simply is not possible for the children to perform barefooted, as when a child is wearing tights, health regulations forbid it, or the floor is dirty or splintered. If the child is wearing tights and the choice becomes sneakers or stocking feet, then choose the sneakers. It is much too dangerous to move in socks or tights even on a carpet, and sensing how easy it would be to slip will greatly restrict the child's freedom of movement.

Teaching Methods

This book employs two of the three teaching methods most often employed in movement education: the *direct approach*, which should play the largest role with this age group, and *exploration*.

THE DIRECT APPROACH Modeling is often the best means to achieve success with toddlers and some children with special needs. As children mature, they have to learn to follow directions and to imitate physically what their eyes are seeing (for example, when they must write the letters of the alphabet as seen in a book or on a board). According to Mosston and Ashworth, "Emulating, repeating, copying, and responding to directions seem to be necessary ingredients of the early years" (1990, 45). They cite Simon Says, Follow the Leader, and songs accompanied by unison clapping or movement as examples of "command-style" activities enjoyed by young children. Mirroring and fingerplays are among the other activities that they suggest fit into the same category.

With the direct approach, the teacher makes all or most of the decisions regarding what, how, and when the children are to perform (Gallahue and Cleland Donnelly 2003). This task-oriented approach requires the teacher to provide a brief explanation, often followed by a demonstration, of what is expected. The children then perform accordingly, usually by imitating what was demonstrated.

One advantage of this approach is that it produces immediate results. This in turn means you can instantly ascertain if a child is having difficulty following directions or producing the required response. For example, if the class is playing Simon Says and a child repeatedly touches the incorrect body part, you are made aware of a potential problem, possibly with hearing, processing information, or simply identifying body parts.

Mosston and Ashworth cite achieving conformity and uniformity as two of the behavior objectives—and perpetuating traditional rituals as one of the subject matter objectives—of the direct approach (1990). For example, if "rituals" like the ones performed to the song "Where Is Thumbkin?" are to be performed in a traditional manner, with all the children doing the same thing at the same time, the only expedient way to facilitate these activities is with a direct approach, using demonstration and imitation. Although conformity and uniformity are not conducive to creativity and self-expression, they are necessary to the performance of certain activities. Because such activities are fun for young children and can produce a sense of belonging, they should play a role in the movement program.

EXPLORATION Exploration is developmentally appropriate for young children and therefore should be widely used in movement programs. Because it results in a *variety* of responses to each challenge presented, it is also known as divergent problem solving. For example, a challenge to demonstrate crooked shapes could result in as many different crooked shapes as there are children responding.

This approach to instruction has never been better described than by Elizabeth Halsey and Lorena Porter:

> [Movement exploration] should follow such basic procedures as: (1) setting the problem; (2) experimentation by the children; (3) observation and evaluation; (4) additional practice using points gained from evaluation. Answers to the problems, of course, are in movements rather than words. The movements will differ as individual children find the answer valid for each. The teacher does not demonstrate, encourage imitation, nor require any one best answer. Thus the children are not afraid to be different, and the teacher feels free to let them progress in their own way, each at his own rate. The result is a class atmosphere in which imagination has free play; invention becomes active and varied. (1970, 76)

In other words, you will present your children with a challenge (for example, "Show me how tall you can be"), and the children will offer their responses in movement. You can then issue additional challenges to continue with and vary the exploration (*extending* the activity), or you can issue follow-up questions and challenges intended to improve or correct what you have seen (*refining* responses).

Extending exploration is a technique that requires time, patience, and practice by the teacher. When teachers are not yet comfortable with all aspects of exploration, they may hurry from one movement challenge to the next. Not only does this leave the class with too much time and nothing left to do, but also it fails to give children ample experience with the exploration process and with the movements being explored.

In addition to issuing a follow-up to "find another way," you can use the elements of movement (considered adverbs used to modify the skills, which are regarded as verbs) to extend activities. For instance, if the locomotor skill of walking were being explored, there would be a number of choices with regard to *how* to perform the walking: forward, backward, to the side, or possibly in a circle. The element of space is being used here. The walk could be performed with arms or head held in various positions (shape), quickly or slowly (time), strongly or lightly (force), with interruptions (flow), or to altering rhythms (rhythm).

Of course, you must design problems and suggest extensions that are developmentally appropriate and relevant to the subject matter and to the children's lives. You must also provide the encouragement children need to continue producing divergent responses. Encouragement should consist of neutral feedback, for example, "I see you're walking in a bent-over shape."

Although you must be careful to accept all responses, there will come a time when you wish to help the children improve, or refine, their solutions. If, for example, you have challenged the children to make themselves as small as possible and some children respond by lying flat on the floor, you should not observe aloud that this response is incorrect.

In fact, it is not necessarily incorrect; it is simply another way of looking at things. However, because you want the children to truly experience a small shape, you might use the follow-up question, "Is there a way you can be small in a very rounded shape?" to encourage a different response. Although you have helped the children improve their responses, individuality is not stifled, as diverse solutions are still possible (for example, some children will make a small rounded shape in a sitting position, some will lie on their backs, others on their sides, and so on).

Adapting Activities

Although movement experiences entail an additional challenge for children with special needs, movement education is well suited to these children. Its philosophy and practice lend themselves to the inclusion of—and success for—all children. Thus, when incorporating children with special needs into movement activities, you must be sure that your challenges can be met by all of the children.

Keep in mind that every child will be able to respond in some manner. For example, Samuelson explained that the blink of an eye, the inhalation of a breath, and the twitching of fingers are all movements (1981). Thus, they can be considered responses to challenges and can even be used for demonstration purposes, with the remaining children being asked to replicate these movements. Not only does this include the child with special needs, but it also places her in what is probably an unfamiliar role—that of leader.

This book, of course, cannot do justice to the vast topic of children with special needs or cover all the different special needs that teachers and caregivers may encounter. However, the following are some guidelines for helping children with physical challenges, hearing impairments, and visual impairments achieve success.

PHYSICAL CHALLENGES In general, the child with physical disabilities should be encouraged to participate at whatever level is possible. A child may have to substitute swaying or nodding the head for more difficult rhythmic responses. If the child cannot hold rhythm instruments, he can wear bells attached to elastics or Velcro placed around his wrists and simply *become* a musical instrument. Children in wheelchairs will have to experience locomotion on wheels rather than on foot—whether propelling themselves or being pushed by a peer. Cane or crutch tapping can substitute for hand clapping or foot stomping, and upper-body movements can replace lower-body movements.

Movement is typically not a problem for children with hearing impairments unless there is damage to the semicircular canals. If so, the children will have balance problems, which can result in delays in motor ability. Children with such damage should refrain from taking part in potentially dangerous balance activities—for example, climbing or tumbling actions requiring rotation—unless assistance is provided.

AUDITORY CHALLENGES For all children with hearing impairments, the major challenges involved in participating in movement experiences are related to the use of music and the presentation of instructions. You can take a number of steps to help lessen the latter problem. Place children with difficulty hearing in the front of the room. Distractions like background music or others talking should be eliminated. When speaking, you should always face the child with a hearing impairment and avoid covering your mouth. You should also speak in low tones (not low as opposed to loud but low as opposed to high pitched) because children with hearing impairments are better able to hear low-frequency sounds. Flicking the lights off and on is a signal that you can use to instantly get children's attention.

During music activities, remember that although a child may not be able to hear the music, she will be able to feel it. Children with hearing impairments can place their hands on the CD player or the instrument being used to make music to feel the vibrations and establish a rhythm. Lying on a wooden floor often enables children to feel the vibrations with the whole body.

Imitation is another important tool in being able to experience rhythms with and without music. Children with hearing impairments should be encouraged to imitate their peers as they clap hands, stamp feet, march, gallop, and skip.

Finally, movement experiences that meet the needs of children at all levels of ability only need minor modifications to meet the needs of children who are visually challenged. Children with visual limitations tend to rely more heavily on adults than do sighted children and often display hesitation and caution when asked to move. However, they have to their advantage auditory and tactile skills that become increasingly stronger, and these senses can be used to enhance kinesthetic skills.

VISUAL CHALLENGES When working with children with visual impairments, you have a number of methods you can use to help ensure greater success. Children with poor vision should be placed near you so they can see more easily. Holding hands with you or with a responsible partner—or having a partner place his hands on the hips or shoulders of the child with visual problems—are ways of using the tactile and kinesthetic senses to encourage movement and alleviate the fear. You can also use touch to help a child achieve an appropriate shape or position.

To make use of the auditory sense, use verbal cues and clear, succinct descriptions when presenting challenges and when offering feedback. Statements like "You are lifting and lowering your heels to move up and down" have the additional benefit of increasing the child's body awareness. Such statements as "Everyone tilt their head side to side" help the visually impaired child realize that her body is like the other children's.

No matter what special needs a child may have, he or she can be included successfully in most movement activities.

Making Transitions

Whether the children are going on to another content area, to lunch, or home to parents at the end of your movement activities, it is always a good idea to help them wind down a bit before sending them on their way. This is where some relaxation techniques come into play.

You may be surprised to learn that relaxation plays other important roles in movement experiences than just offering rest. Relaxation prepares children for slow or sustained movement, which requires greater control than fast movement. Being relaxed also provides children with the opportunity to experience motionlessness, giving more meaning, in contrast, to movement.

Tension control can also help children learn better, as stress has been shown to have a negative impact on learning. Furthermore, if you use imagery to promote relaxation, you will be enhancing the children's ability to imagine. If you use music, you will be exposing the children to the world of quiet, serene music. The following are some specific suggestions.

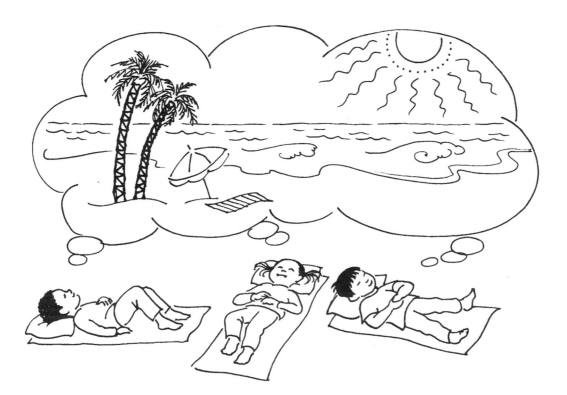

IMAGERY What comes to mind when you think of rag dolls, limp noodles, melting ice cubes, or soggy dishrags? Relaxation! (Whenever possible, *show* toddlers examples of what you want them to emulate.) Ask the children to pretend to be one of these objects, and just watch those muscles relax. Or paint a picture in their minds: Ask them to lie on the floor, imagining they are floating on a cloud or at the beach. For the latter, you might talk to them (softly!) about the warmth of the sun, the cool breeze, and the gentle sounds of the waves and the gulls circling overhead; and do not be surprised if a few of them drop off to sleep.

SLEEPING CONTEST If you have a particularly competitive—or active—group of children, you might find that a sleeping contest works best of all. Ask them to show you who in the class can sleep the soundest (without snoring!), and just watch as they drop to the floor! Of course, there can be no one winner, so you'll have to congratulate them all on being the best sleeping class you have ever seen.

MUSIC There are many soothing pieces to choose from, whether with vocals or without—including classical music from the distant past (Mozart, Bach, and Chopin wrote some wonderfully soothing pieces) as well as New Age music, lullabies, or some of the many children's recordings made specifically for "quiet times."

Teaching Hints

The following suggestions are offered to help you facilitate movement experiences as smoothly as possible:

- Always familiarize yourself with a lesson or activity, and particularly with a song, *before* trying it with the children.
- When an activity calls for music, the lesson plan will specify this with a musical note (♪) and indicate which song on the accompanying CD is to be used. The Song List will also help you find the song you need.
- Discuss new or unfamiliar words or images from songs or poems with the children prior to the activity.
- It may be helpful to first allow children to *listen* to a new song— with or without lyrics—before asking them to move to it.

- Introduce each activity to the children ("Now we're going to explore *up* and *down*").
- Always be sure children are both familiar and comfortable with an activity before trying its extensions.
- The lesson plans leave plenty of room for your personality and imagination. Please feel free to use them!

Toddlers: Developmental Considerations

The following is some information concerning the characteristics and development of children ages eighteen to thirty-six months. Some of these facts are ones you are already aware of and serve here as reminders. Together with the others, they will give you a better idea of what you can expect from your children as you begin this program.

- Morning is the best time for toddlers to participate in movement. If afternoon is your only option, wait until the children have been up from their naps for a while before expecting them to be creative.
- You will need a great deal of time to organize toddlers as a group. Thus, it would be impractical to plan to spend fewer than twenty minutes per movement session.
- Toddlers are a restless lot. You probably should not plan to hold their attention for longer than thirty minutes!
- The more individual attention you can give to a toddler during movement exploration, the better. The general rule is to have no more than five toddlers per adult.
- Verbalization and visual aids can be extremely helpful when exploring movement with very young children, especially where imagery is concerned. If you want the children to adopt the shape of a ball, show them a ball or a picture of one. If you are going to ask them to move the way dogs move, talk to them first about canine characteristics.

- The development of gross (large-muscle) motor skills will occur according to each child's individual timetable. By three years of age, however, children usually have good large-muscle control.
- At the toddler stage, jumping will most likely be executed from a flat-footed stance with the body weight shifted backward. It is only after children become more proficient at the flat-footed jump that they can begin a jump from the balls of the feet, swinging the arms forward and upward and finally shifting body weight forward. Also, toddlers tend to land with their knees straight and on one foot before the other.
- Balancing skills will, of course, be wobbly in the beginning. At first the children will require greater use of their arms, even for static balances—balances achieved while remaining in one spot. However, as your toddlers become more secure (for example, less afraid of losing their balance), they will also display more steadiness with less effort.

The following are some other general milestones that normally take place by certain ages.

By age two, a child should be able to do the following:

- jump in place
- jump from a bottom step

By age two and a half, a child should be able to do the following:

- long jump approximately twenty-four to thirty-four inches
- balance on one foot for one second
- take four steps on tiptoe

By age three, a child should be able to do the following:

- walk on tiptoe for ten feet
- balance on one foot for five seconds

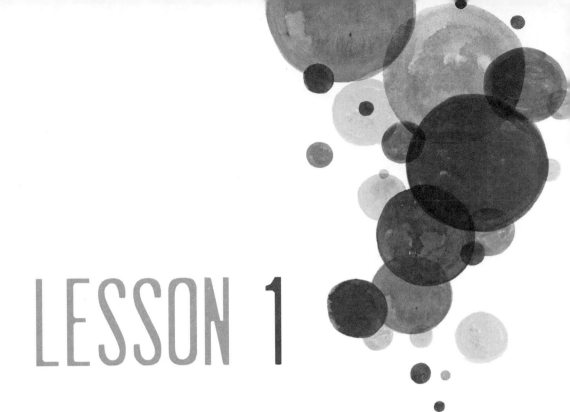

LESSON 1

Heads, Bellies, Toes

Ask the children to touch their heads, bellies, and toes, and then reverse the order as you call out the body parts. Begin with a slow, rhythmic chant that gently moves the children down and up. Once the children are experiencing success with this, reverse—and mix up—the order of body parts.

Extending the Activity: Vary the tempo at which you call out the body parts, or start out slowly and gradually accelerate (*the movement element of time*). Add dramatic pauses—long and short—so the children are not sure when you will call out a body part (*flow*).

When your toddlers are ready, play the more traditional Heads, Shoulders, Knees, and Toes, eventually varying the order of body parts and the tempo at which you call them out.

Observation and Evaluation: Can the child identify body parts? Does the child demonstrate listening skills?

Adding Equipment: Children can touch plastic cups, rhythm sticks, or beanbags to the body parts instead of their hands to provide practice manipulating an object.

Curriculum Connectors: Body-part identification is an important introductory concept for young children, falling under the theme of "My Body" and the content area of *science*. Listening skills are a component of both *language arts* and *music*.

Let's Stretch

Stretching is always a good exercise, whether it is the arms, legs, or trunk doing the stretching. Lead the children in a little of each, remembering to stretch forward, backward, toward the ceiling, and toward the floor. (*Note:* Knees should always be slightly bent when stretching toward the floor.)

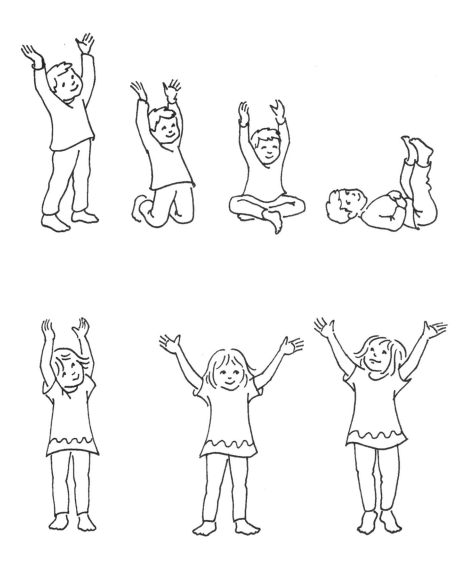

Extending the Activity: The next step is to simply issue the challenges and let the children respond in their own ways. Ask your toddlers to do these movements:

- reach for the ceiling
- kneel and stretch ("How many ways can you stretch while kneeling?")
- sit and stretch
- lie on the back and stretch the legs toward the ceiling
- crouch low and then stretch up quickly, like a jack-in-the-box popping up
- stretch bodies high while the arms stretch low

Observation and Evaluation: Is the child able to stretch body parts in each of the directions presented? Does the child bend knees slightly when stretching forward at the waist?

Curriculum Connectors: Stretching muscles falls under the heading of *science*, and contributes to flexibility, one of the health-related components of physical fitness. The directional concepts are relative to *art*, but they are also prepositions (*language arts*) and are central to early geometry (*mathematics*).

Let's Walk

 "Walking Along" (Length 1:51)—CD Track 1

Easing into the transitions as gently as possible, encourage the children to do the following, allowing them plenty of time to fully explore each challenge.

Ask your toddlers to walk in these ways:

- freely (with good posture—"Nice and tall.")
- in place ("Show me you can make your knees go higher. Go a little faster.")
- forward ("Can you do it slower?")
- backward (carefully, for just a few steps!)
- as tall as possible
- as small as possible

Extending the Activity: Have the children experiment with the listed ways of walking while "Walking Along" is played. Feel free to include any other walking ideas that the music inspires. Please do not fret if the toddlers do not perform these activities in time with the beat of the music. That will come with practice.

Generally speaking, you can expect your toddlers to take about four steps on tiptoe by the time they reach twenty-seven months. When you feel they are ready, increase the challenge by inviting the children to give walking on tiptoe a try.

To incorporate imagery into the locomotor skill of walking, discuss the following images with your toddlers, and then ask them to walk like they are the following:

- big and strong
- fat and jolly like Santa Claus
- really mad
- really sad
- trying to find a towel with soap in their eyes
- in a parade
- trying to get through sticky mud

Observation and Evaluation: Does the child demonstrate proper posture and alignment, with weight distributed evenly over all five toes and the heel of the foot? Does the child respond appropriately to the imagery used?

Adding Equipment: Play "Walking Along," inviting the children to accompany the song with rhythm instruments. Those not developmentally ready to walk and play an instrument at the same time should be allowed to simply stand and play.

Curriculum Connectors: By accompanying the activity with "Walking Along," you are bringing in the content area of *music*. Because self-discovery, including the exploration of emotions, is the first step in *social studies* for young children, using the suggested imagery incorporates that content area. Directional concepts are essential to reading and writing (*language arts*).

Exploring Up and Down

Ask the children whether they know what *up* and *down* mean, and to show you with their bodies. Then pose the following questions and movement challenges:

- Can you make your body go all the way down? Can you go all the way up?
- How high up can you get?
- Go down halfway. What does that mean to you?
- Make yourself so tiny I can hardly see you.
- Make yourself as huge as a giant.

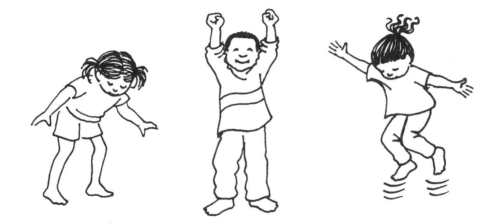

Extending the Activity: Play a game of Blast Off. Ask your toddlers to squat down, pretending to be rockets on launching pads. You then count down from ten (with as much drama as possible!), and at the signal to "blast off," the children spring up and "into the air." Your toddlers will love this, so you should expect to have to repeat it at least a few times!

You can also use imagery to explore the concepts of up and down. Talk about the following, and then ask your toddlers to show you these objects:

- a piece of bread going in and then popping out of the toaster
- a yo-yo on a string
- a jack-in-the-box (first being pushed down and then springing up)
- popcorn popping (starting with little kernels in the pan)

Observation and Evaluation: Does the child demonstrate understanding of the concepts involved? Is the child able to relate to the imagery used?

Adding Equipment: Invite the children to experiment with moving a scarf or balloon up and down. Although this can be an introduction to the manipulative skills of throwing, catching, and volleying, you should simply allow the children to explore the possibilities on their own.

Curriculum Connectors: The levels in space—low, middle, and high—are quantitative concepts falling under the heading of *mathematics* and spatial concepts falling under *art*.

LESSON 2

Show Me

Explain to the children that you want to see how well they know their body parts, so they should point to, touch, or display the part when they hear you call out its name. You can ask the children to show you a variety of body parts, including the following:

nose	knees
toes	tummies
eyes	mouth
hands	tongue
ears	shoulders

Extending the Activity: Once you have addressed these familiar body parts, move on to more challenging parts, like chins, hips, elbows, wrists, ankles, and temples.

Observation and Evaluation: Can the child identify body parts? Does the child demonstrate listening skills?

Adding Equipment: Provide the children with chiffon scarves, challenging them to balance the scarf on a variety of body parts, first while remaining in one spot, and later while traveling. Scarves can most easily be balanced on the hand and the top of the head. But do not rule out the nose, forearm, or shoulder. When the children are ready for a greater challenge, provide them with beanbags to balance on body parts.

Curriculum Connectors: Body-part identification is an important introductory concept for young children, falling under the theme of "My Body" and the content area of *science*, as does the concept of balance.

Let's Bend

Explain to the children that bending is another way of exploring up and down. Then ask them to do these movements:

- bend forward; backward; to the side
- touch their knees and straighten
- touch their toes and straighten very slowly
- touch their toes and straighten halfway

Extending the Activity: Follow this by asking the children to experiment with bending the waist, arms, and legs while kneeling, crouching, sitting, and lying on backs, stomachs, and sides. Are there other body parts they can find that bend? (Possibilities include fingers, neck, and ankles.)

Observation and Evaluation: Is the child able to bend the appropriate body parts in the directions given? Does the child demonstrate understanding of the concept of bending?

Curriculum Connectors: To make *mathematics* part of the activity, challenge the children to count how many ways different parts can bend. For instance, a knee can only bend one way, but you can bend at the waist in four different directions. Identifying and exploring how body parts function is *science*.

Let's Run

 "The Track Meet" (Length 1:04)—CD Track 2

Toddlers love to run! However, for this activity you should stress safety and the fact that they are going to try running in different ways. Ask the children to run in the following ways:

- in place ("Show me you can make your knees go higher. Go a little faster. Now slower.")
- forward, making a lot of noise with the feet
- very lightly, with tiny steps
- on signal and stop; run again
- following the leader (you) in straight, curving, and zigzag paths

Extending the Activity: Have the children experiment with running while "The Track Meet" plays. They can pretend they are jogging around a track, or you can use some of the above examples to vary the ways in which they are running.

Another option is to play a game of Make-Believe Running, in which you incorporate imagery into the exploration of this locomotor skill. Talk to the children about the images below and then ask them to pretend to run, with or without the music, as though

carrying a ball	in a race
on very hot sand that	bouncing a ball
is burning their feet	very tired

Observation and Evaluation: Does the child demonstrate good posture and proper alignment, with weight evenly distributed over all five toes and the heel of the foot? Does the child use limbs in opposition (for example, left arm and right leg forward, then right arm and left leg forward)? Does the child respond to the imagery used?

Curriculum Connectors: Use of the song incorporates *music*. The use of such terms as *higher*, *faster*, and *slower* promotes emergent literacy (*language arts*).

Exploring Straight and Round

Talk about *straight* and *round* with the children, showing them examples or pictures of these shapes, discussing how they differ from one another. What other things can they think of that are either straight or round? Then ask them if they can show you the following with their bodies:

Straight	Round
a ruler	a pancake
a wall	a ball
a pencil	a Frisbee

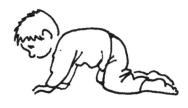 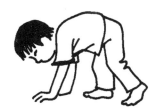 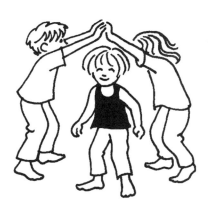

Extending the Activity: Ask the children to show you straight and round in the following ways:

- standing
- way up high
- kneeling
- sitting
- lying on the floor
- with their arms
- with their legs

Following these experiences with straight and round, the children should be ready to demonstrate bridges and tunnels. Show them pictures of bridges and tunnels, discussing how they are similar to and differ from one another. Then ask them to show you both with their bodies. Can they make the bridge look different from the tunnel? To make the activity more challenging, ask them to show you how many body parts can create bridges and tunnels. Or have them form tunnels in pairs, with a third child going through the "structure."

Observation and Evaluation: Does the child understand the concepts of *straight* and *round*? Is the child able to physically demonstrate them? Is the child able to respond to the images of bridges and tunnels?

Curriculum Connectors: Shape is a concept critical to both *art* and *mathematics*. The topic of bridges and tunnels falls under the theme of transportation, which belongs to the content area of *social studies*.

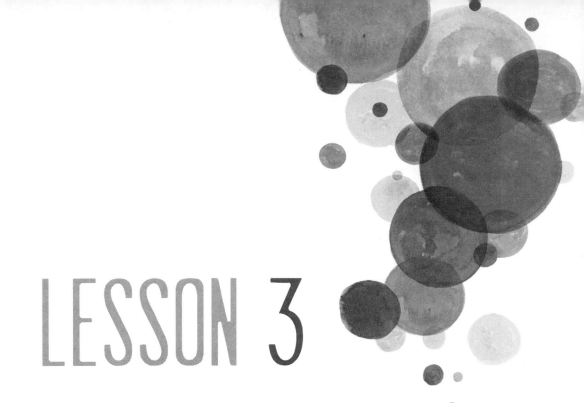

LESSON 3

Flexing/Pointing Feet

Sit with the children on the floor, either with your legs straight out in front or in a straddle position, and demonstrate what it looks like to point and flex the feet. Ask the children to first point and flex both together. Then, when they are comfortable with this, have them point one foot at a time, alternating right and left. (*Note:* Toddlers also love to say the words *point* and *flex*, so encourage them to call out the words along with the actions!)

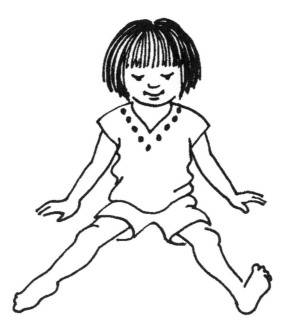

Extending the Activity: Talk to the children about all the different things their feet help them do, and then ask them to show you how they move when they do these things. Possibilities include:

walking	climbing stairs
running	kicking a ball
skating	stamping
jumping	dancing

Observation and Evaluation: Is the child able to point and flex feet simultaneously and then alternately? Can the child demonstrate the motor skills cited?

Adding Equipment: Give the children each a beanbag to manipulate around the floor with their feet. A beanbag is much easier to control than a ball, so it will provide a wonderful introductory experience to the manipulative skill of dribbling.

Curriculum Connectors: To incorporate *language arts*, accompany the pointing and flexing activity with the following rhyme:

Point and flex
And circle my feet.
Put them together and
The bottoms meet!

Let's Shake

♪ **"Wiggle, Wiggle, Shake and Giggle" (Length 1:22)—CD Track 3**

Sit with the children and explore the nonlocomotor skill of shaking by shaking one or both hands in front of the body, at either side, up high, and down low. Then pose the following challenges:

- Show me you can find another part of your body to shake.
- Stand and find parts of your body to shake.
- Shake your whole body all at once.

Extending the Activity: Now that you have explored shaking with the children, wiggling and giggling should be no problem! Move with the children to "Wiggle, Wiggle, Shake and Giggle." The lyrics are as follows:

Wiggle like a worm.
Wiggle like a snake.
Then wind it up
And shake, shake, shake!
Wiggle a little,
Now wiggle a lot.

Then stay right there
And shake in your spot!
Let's see a wiggle.
Let's see a shake.
Now it's time to
Take a giggle break!

Observation and Evaluation: Is the child able to shake various body parts? Does the child differentiate between shaking and wiggling?

Adding Equipment: If you have maracas or other shaking instruments available, pass them out and let the children *hear* the sound of shaking and wiggling!

Curriculum Connectors: Using the song is a way to incorporate both *language arts* and *music*.

Let's Jump

♪ **"Rabbits and 'Roos" (Length 1:02)—CD Track 4**

A jump propels the body upward from a takeoff on two feet. The toes, which are the last to leave the ground (heel-ball-toe), are the first to reach it upon landing, with landings occurring toe-ball-heel and with knees bent.

Although you certainly cannot expect this kind of execution from your toddlers, children are generally able to jump in place by the time they are twenty-three months old. Show your children what a jump looks like, and then ask them to try it for themselves. How many can they do in a row? How high off the floor can they get?

Extending the Activity: Present the following challenges:

- Jump with your feet barely coming off the floor. Try it with your feet coming way off.
- Show me you can make your knees go higher.
- Jump, being as tall (small) as you can be.
- Jump forward, toward that wall (column, desk, and so on) over there.
- Show me you can jump in a circle.
- Show me you can jump fast. Slowly.

Talk to your toddlers about rabbits and kangaroos, showing pictures if you have them available. Discuss the fact that they both jump as a way of getting around, but that kangaroos are much bigger, so their jumps are much heavier than the rabbits' jumps.

Play "Rabbits and 'Roos," and invite the children to move like rabbits during the A section and like kangaroos during the B section. (Don't worry if the children choose not to jump despite your discussion; just so long as they are pretending to be the animal.) The form of the song is ABAB (rabbits, 'roos, rabbits, 'roos).

Observation and Evaluation: Does the child use the legs and toes to execute a jump? Does the child land with heels coming all the way to the floor, with knees bent? Does the child demonstrate understanding of the movement elements involved?

Curriculum Connectors: Using the song encompasses *music*, while exploring animal movements falls under the heading of *science*. Also, *light* and *heavy* are quantitative concepts falling under the content area of *mathematics*.

Shapes in Motion

Tell the children you are all going to walk around the room together. Explain that every once in a while you are going to change the shape of your body, and that each child should try to make the same shape with his or her body. Possible shapes can include these:

- arms out to the side
- arms above head
- hands on hips
- head tilted to one (or the other) side
- crouching

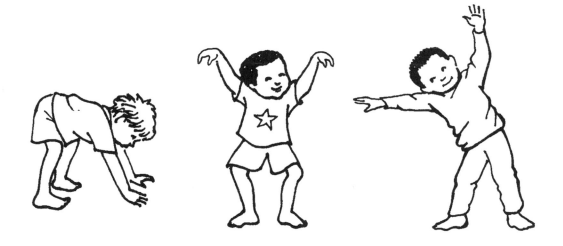

Extending the Activity: To further the challenge, stand before the children, assuming shapes the children can try to duplicate. This gives you more leeway with regard to the shapes you make, but you may want to preface each shape with a brief description (for example, "Kneeling," "On tiptoe," and so on), making verbalization a part of the activity. Suggestions for shapes include the following:

on tiptoe   hands on hips

with arms above head or out to sides   kneeling

bent at the waist   sitting

bent at the knees

The children have experimented with a variety of shapes at this point and have had the opportunity to explore round and straight shapes. For this activity, you should review *round* and *straight* and follow that up with a discussion of the other shapes the children can try to show you here. Then ask them to show you bodies that have these shapes:

round	long	crooked
straight	short	wide
flat		

Can they also show you the shapes of these familiar items with their bodies?

tree	teapot	ball
table	pencil	rug

Observation and Evaluation: Is the child able to physically replicate what the eyes are seeing? Can the child demonstrate the appropriate shapes?

Adding Equipment: Give each child a jump rope. Invite the children to make a shape on the floor with the rope, and then imitate the shape or follow its path by walking along it.

Curriculum Connectors: Shape is integral to both *mathematics* and *art*. Also integral to art and to writing (*language arts*) is the ability to physically replicate what the eyes see.

LESSON 4

Where Is Thumbkin?

♪ **"Where Is Thumbkin?" (Length 2:07)—CD Track 5**

This old standard is performed in the usual manner, asking the whereabouts of thumbkin, pointer, middle finger, ring finger, baby finger, and the whole family (with the fingers hiding behind the back until the response "Here I am" is to be sung). However, in this version the lyrics are missing where the responses should be, allowing the children to sing the responses themselves while displaying the appropriate finger. In response to "Where is . . . ?" the children sing, "Here I am, here I am." To the question "How are you this fine day?" they respond, "Very well, I thank you" (the appropriate finger on one hand asks the question and the other responds).

Extending the Activity: Ask the children to make a fist. Then, as you very slowly count 1-2-3-4-5, have them display their fingers, one at a time. Then reverse, counting backward, with the children "closing" one finger at a time. Repeat a few more times, gradually increasing the tempo. (*Note:* This may be hard for some to coordinate, but assure them it will come with practice.)

Observation and Evaluation: Does the child participate by singing and with actions? Does the child display the appropriate finger(s)? Is the child able to open and close the fingers?

Curriculum Connectors: The song offers children experience with *music*, while the lyrics and fine-motor skills incorporate *language arts*. The counting in the extension activity falls under the heading of *mathematics*.

Let's Sway

♪ **"The Swaying Song" (Length 1:27)—CD Track 6**

A *sway* transfers weight from one part of the body to another in an easy, relaxed motion. Demonstrate swaying to the children, and then ask them to try it, both side to side and front to back. (*Note:* Although you can point out that the toes at least should remain on the floor, you can probably expect the children to lift their feet entirely at this point.)

Extending the Activity: To make this activity more challenging, invite children to stand in a circle, swaying while holding hands or with hands on one another's shoulders. Later, if you feel they are ready, ask them to sway with arms around one another's waists or shoulders. Practice all of this to the accompaniment of "The Swaying Song" to give them the appropriate "feel."

Observation and Evaluation: Does the child understand the concept of swaying? Is the child able to execute the skill? Does the child move cooperatively with others?

Adding Equipment: Chiffon scarves, streamers, and ribbon sticks are props that lend themselves beautifully to the nonlocomotor skill of swaying—and can sometimes help children understand how the movement should look and feel.

Curriculum Connectors: Swaying is a basic example of balance and recovery, which is a concept falling under simple *science*. Using the song incorporates *music*.

Tiny Steps/Giant Steps

Establish an audible signal with the children (for example, two hand claps, a tap on the drum). Then instruct them to move with tiny steps until they hear the signal, at which time they begin taking giant steps. Continue to alternate, varying the amount of time they have to perform each.

Extending the Activity: Read this poem in its entirety, explaining anything you feel needs clarification, such as the difference between very big and very small. Then read it aloud again, moving with the children and pretending to be giants and elves.

See the giants, great and tall.
Hear them bellow, hear them call.
Life looks different from up so high,
With head and shoulders clear to the sky.
And at their feet they can barely see
The little people so very tiny,
Who scurry about with hardly a care

Avoiding enormous feet placed here and
  there.
But together they dwell, the giants and
  elves,
In peace and harmony, amongst
  themselves.

Observation and Evaluation: Does the child differentiate between tiny steps and giant steps? Does the child understand the concepts of giants (very big people) and elves (very tiny people)?

Curriculum Connectors: The concepts of *length* and *size* are important to both *mathematics* and *art*. Also, the quantitative concepts in the poem (for example, *high*, *together*) offer more experience with math. Using the poem incorporates *language arts*, as does experience with the opposites of *enormous* and *tiny*.

Up and Down Make-Believe

Ask the children to imagine they are each a brightly colored balloon (in the color of their choice!). Then demonstrate how they can look like inflating balloons by starting in a small shape and slowly growing bigger while inhaling through the nose. To depict a deflating balloon, they slowly decrease in size while exhaling through the mouth. (*Note:* Repeat this only once or twice to avoid hyperventilation.)

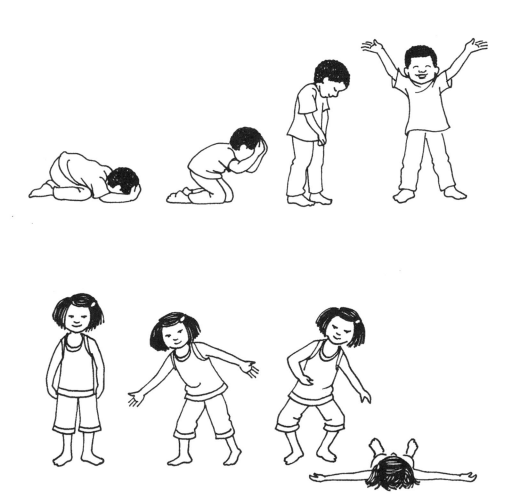

Extending the Activity: Once children have demonstrated an ability to remain in one spot and move slowly, talk to them about seeds growing and ice cubes melting, again emphasizing *slow* movement. Then ask them to get down on the floor and into the smallest shapes possible, imagining that they are tiny little seeds planted in the earth. After some rain and sunshine, which you can "provide" if you like, they begin to grow very slowly; and they continue to grow until they are the biggest and best flowers and trees ever.

Now ask them to imagine they have suddenly turned into giant ice cubes. When the sun shines on them, they start, ever so slowly, to melt—until they are nothing but puddles of water on the ground!

Observation and Evaluation: Is the child able to move slowly? Does the child respond to the imagery involved? Does the child understand the concepts of *up* and *down*, *big* and *small*?

Adding Equipment: Demonstrating with an actual balloon can help toddlers to better understand the concepts of slow inflation and deflation. (*Note:* Because of the potential choking hazard, the teacher should keep the balloon within her reach at all times.)

Curriculum Connectors: Inflation and deflation, seeds growing, and ice cubes melting are all concepts falling under the heading of *science*. Size, position, and time are *mathematics* concepts.

LESSON 5

Open and Close

· ·

♪ **"Open and Close" (Length 1:34)—CD Track 7**

The words to this song are self-explanatory, but you may want to first review them as a poem. Whether you use the words as a poem or a song, show the children how to act out each line.

These are the lyrics:

Open your eyes, close your eyes,
Open them up again!
Now close them tight with all your might—
As tight as you can, and then
Open your hands, close your hands,
Open them up again!
Now close them tight with all your might—
As tight as you can, and then
Open your mouth, close your mouth,

Open it up again!
Now close it tight with all your might—
As tight as you can, and then
Open your arms, close your arms,
Open them up again!
Now close them tight with all your might—
And you're hugging your best friend—
Hugging your best friend!

Extending the Activity: Challenge your toddlers to experiment with closing and opening such body parts as feet, knees, legs, wrists, and elbows. What would it look like to "close" and "open" the whole body? Can they do it slowly? Quickly? Light as a feather?

Observation and Evaluation: Can the child identify body parts? Can the child demonstrate the concepts of *open* and *close*?

Adding Equipment: Opening and closing the body and body parts can be even more fun while encased in or holding on to Body Sox (available from physical education suppliers) or stretchy fabric (either large enough for one child at a time or for a small group of children).

Curriculum Connectors: Body-part identification can be classified as *science* for young children, as can the concepts of opening and closing. "Open and Close" contributes to both *music* and *language arts*.

Let's Turn

Children love to turn themselves around, and even to make themselves dizzy, which is actually a good balance exercise. In this activity, however, they will be introduced to the nonlocomotor skill of turning as a *controlled* skill—a rotation of the body around an axis that can occur in a great variety of ways.

Pose the following challenges:

- Show me you can stay in your space and turn yourself gently around in one direction.
- Now go the other way.
- Turn yourself around very, very slowly.
- Turn with your arms out to your sides.
- Now turn with your arms over your head.
- Turn around quickly—once.

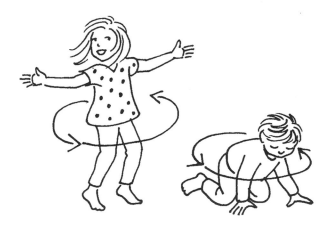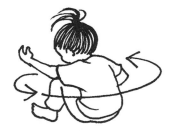

Extending the Activity: To make this skill more challenging for your toddlers, ask them to turn in the following ways:

- while being as tall (small) as they can
- while on knees (one knee)
- while sitting on their bottoms
- while on one (the other) foot

(*Note:* Though the latter may prove to be too challenging for some toddlers, they will still find it fun to try.)

Observation and Evaluation: Is the child able to turn while remaining in one spot? Does the child demonstrate good balance? How many of the challenges can the child manage successfully?

Adding Equipment: Asking each child to execute these tasks while standing inside a plastic hoop or on a poly spot can help with the concept of remaining in place.

Curriculum Connectors: Directionality is essential to success in reading and writing (*language arts*). To add *music* and more language arts components to the activity, sing the following to the tune of "Old McDonald Had a Farm."

I can turn myself around;
Watch me go this way.
Now watch me turn myself around
In the other way.
I can turn fast; I can turn slow.
I can turn many ways, you know.
I can turn myself around
With both feet on the ground.

Let's Gallop

A gallop is a locomotor skill that differs from the walk and the run in that it is performed with an uneven rhythm. It is a combination of a walk and a leap in which one foot leads and the other plays catch-up. Most children can gallop by the time they are three, but to ensure success for *all* your toddlers, simply suggest that they pretend to be horses. Since galloping is a skill often learned by imitation, you should pretend to be a horse too!

Extending the Activity: When children have mastered galloping with the preferred (easier) foot leading, suggest they at least *try* it with the nonpreferred (more difficult) foot leading.

Observation and Evaluation: Is the child able to execute a gallop with the preferred foot leading? Does the back foot play catch-up with, but not pass, the leading foot? Can the child gallop with the other (nonpreferred) foot leading?

Adding Equipment: Using stick horses can help make this locomotor skill easier to learn! It is also helpful to hear the uneven rhythm of a gallop, a cue you can provide with hands, rhythm sticks, or a hand drum.

Curriculum Connectors: Rhythm is a component of both *music* and *language arts*. Focus on the movement of an animal involves *science*.

Pop Goes the Weasel

♪ **"Pop Goes the Weasel" (Length 1:10)—CD Track 8**

Invite the children to crouch in their own spaces, pretending to be a jack-in-the-box that jumps up at the sound of the "pop." Then, once you feel the children are familiar enough with the song, ask them to walk to this familiar melody, jumping lightly into the air each time they hear the "pop."

Extending the Activity: The next step is to ask children to jump into the air and *change direction* at the sound of the "pop." Finally, challenge them to *freeze* at the sound of the pop, moving again only after the song has resumed.

Observation and Evaluation: Does the child exhibit the necessary listening skills? Is the child able to change direction as required? Can the child stop and start on signal?

Curriculum Connectors: Listening is one of the components of *language arts* and is essential in *music*. Directionality is part of both *mathematics* and language arts.

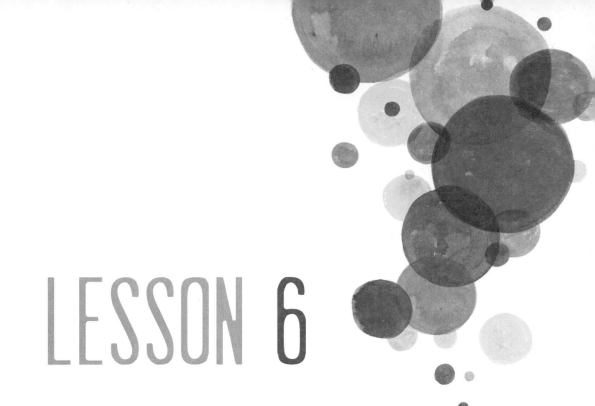

LESSON 6

The Wash Song

♪ "The Wash Song" (Length 1:42)—CD Track 9

Discuss washing, or bathing, with the children, and then tell them this song is going to ask them to pretend to be washing different parts of their bodies. For the last verse, they can pretend to wash a body part of their own choosing (possibilities include leg, back, elbow, foot, chest, arm, shoulder, or neck).

If you like, you can familiarize the children with the song as a poem first. These are the lyrics:

See me wash my face,
From forehead to my chin.
Don't you think my face
Is the best place to begin?
See me wash my hands,
My fingers and my thumbs.
I like to wash my hands.
How clean they have become!
See me wash my tummy,
Around and 'round I go.

When I'm through with my tummy
It will almost glow!
See me wash my knees,
Yes, they're important too.
And now I've done my knees
There's that much less to do!
See me wash my _____,
Yes, I can make it shine.
I can't forget my _____,
Because, you see, it's mine!

Extending the Activity: Challenge children to show you how they would wash such body parts as fingers, toes, heels, ankles, wrists, and temples. Invite them to demonstrate how they would wash their hair. Can they make up a song about brushing hair and/or teeth?

Observation and Evaluation: Is the child developmentally ready to listen and move at the same time? Can the child accurately identify body parts? Does the child contribute suggestions for body parts to wash?

Adding Equipment: Providing each child with a chiffon scarf representing a washcloth can contribute to the fun!

Curriculum Connectors: The primary concept of the song involves hygiene, which, along with body-part identification, falls under the content area of *science*. Of course, the activity also provides experience with *music* and *language arts*.

Bending and Stretching

This activity incorporates imagery into bending and stretching. Ask the children to show you what it looks like to move in these ways:

- Stretch as though you are picking fruit from a tall tree.
- Flop like a rag doll.
- Stretch as though you are waking up and yawning first thing in the morning.
- Bend to tie your shoes.
- Stretch to put something on a high shelf.
- Bend to pat a dog; a cat.
- Stretch to shoot a basketball through a hoop.
- Bend to pick something up from the floor.
- Stretch as though you are climbing a ladder.
- Bend to pick vegetables or flowers from the garden.
- Reach for a star!

Extending the Activity: The following represent more challenging explorations of bending and stretching. If the children are not yet ready to do these stretching motions on their own, model for them.

- Stretch one arm high and the other low.
- Bend one arm while stretching the other one high.
- Reach with both arms to one (the other) side.
- Reach one arm to the side and the other toward the ceiling.
- Bend the knees while stretching arms toward the ceiling.
- Get on hands and knees and stretch one leg (the other) to the back.
- Lie on the back and bend one leg while stretching the other.

Observation and Evaluation: Does the child respond to the imagery involved? Can the child bend and stretch at the same time?

Curriculum Connectors: Bending and stretching are good ways to explore spatial relationships like *up* and *down*, which are important concepts to both *art* and *mathematics*.

Let's Creep

Talk to the children about creeping, explaining that this skill involves moving on hands and knees, or hands and feet, and that babies are not the only creatures that move in this way. Then ask them to creep in the following ways—but if you do not have mats or a carpet to creep on, keep the activity short.

Challenge toddlers to creep in these ways:

- forward slowly
- backward quickly
- as close to the floor as possible in a circle

Extending the Activity: Add imagery to the skill of creeping. Talk to the children about the differences among the following, and ask them to creep like these:

- dog
- cat
- spider
- elephant
- a baby just learning how

Observation and Evaluation: Is the child able to move on hands and knees, or hands and feet, with limbs in opposition? Does the child respond to the concepts and images involved?

Adding Equipment: Providing something for the children to creep through, like tunnels, cut-out foam shapes, or simply large cardboard boxes can help motivate children to keep practicing this important locomotor skill.

Curriculum Connectors: Consideration of how various animals move constitutes *science*. Also, recent brain research indicates that the ability to cross the midline of the body (running from head to feet and separating the body into left and right halves) often connects with the ability to perform cross-lateral movement and contributes to reading and writing abilities (*language arts*).

Moving Slow/Moving Fast

. . . .

♪ "Moving Slow/Moving Fast" (Length 1:26)—CD Track 10

This song focuses on the movement element of time and the musical element of tempo. Play "Moving Slow/Moving Fast," and ask the children to move in whatever way the music makes them feel like moving, or make the following suggestions, one at a time:

Slow	Fast
swaying	tiptoeing
moving like a butterfly	running lightly
soft giant steps	jumping in place

Extending the Activity: Talk to the children about the following images, and then ask them to show them to you. Performing slow and fast in alternation will give toddlers a chance to fully experience the contrast and to acquire the necessary control.

Have the images they demonstrate include these:

a turtle	a rowboat
a rabbit	a jet plane
a worm	an ice cube melting
a bird flying	

Observation and Evaluation: Does the child respond appropriately to the slow and fast tempos of the music? Is the child able to move slowly as well as quickly? Does the child respond to the imagery involved?

Adding Equipment: Providing children with props and asking them to demonstrate how the music makes the *prop* feel like moving often can take the focus off the individual child. It also offers children the opportunity to actually see the difference between slow and fast movement. Streamers and ribbon sticks are great to use with this song.

Curriculum Connectors: Using the song contributes to the children's knowledge of the concept of tempo (*music*). Time is a concept relative to *mathematics*. The alternate activity additionally requires the children to consider both animal movement (*science*) and forms of transportation (*social studies*).

LESSON 7

See My Hands

 "Hands-Hands-Hands" (Length 1:48)—CD Track 11

Ask the children to do the following with you:

- stretch hands and fingers as wide as possible; bend them into tightly clenched fists
- move fingers in and out (start slowly and then increase in tempo)
- bring hands together with lots of force, as though to clap them, but do not let them touch
- repeat, using very little force, so movements are soft and light
- clasp hands together and move them up and down, in and out, and side to side
- turn hands from front to back

Extending the Activity: Because responses can vary depending upon individual imaginations, you should not demonstrate. Instead, merely suggest that the children show these to you:

praying hands	hands directing traffic
hands waving good-bye	patting hands
painting hands	clapping hands

Slowly read the following lyrics aloud as though it were a poem. (*Note:* The words of the poem talk about dialing a phone and putting it back on the hook. You may need to explain about older phones.) Act it out with the children, but encourage them to find their own responses to the question asked in the last two lines:

*Would you like to have some fun with
  your hands?
There are many things they can do.
They can push and pull and lead a band,
And that's just to name a few!*

*They can make fists that shake in the air
When you're mad as you can be.
They reach out to show someone you care
By touching her tenderly.*

A hand is something that bounces a ball
And it turns the page of a book.
It dials the phone when you make a call
And puts it back on the hook!
With your hand you pet your favorite cat
And feel the softness of fur.
It's your hands that hold your baseball bat
And with a spoon help you stir!

Can you show me a drummer when he
  plays
Or somebody scrubbing pans?
Can you think of a few other ways
That you just might use your hands?

Once the children are familiar with "Hands-Hands-Hands" as a poem, try it as a song!

Observation and Evaluation: Can the child imitate your hand motions? Does the child respond appropriately to the imagery involved?

Curriculum Connectors: The identification of body parts—and the exploration of their use—constitutes *science* for young children. Using the lyrics provides experience with *language arts*, while the song brings in *music*.

Let's Strike

A strike is a strong movement of the arm, or arms, propelled in any direction for the purpose of hitting an object. The arm must bend to initiate the strike, extend with both force and speed, and then abruptly stop, with no follow-through in the motion of the arm.

Obviously, before exploring this skill you will have to discuss *pretending* with the toddlers, emphasizing that their strikes are to take place in the air only! Then ask them to strike in the following ways, while standing, kneeling, and sitting:

> with both arms
> with one (the other) arm
> alternating arms
> upward; downward; sideways

Extending the Activity: When your toddlers are ready, challenge them to strike as though they are doing the following:

> playing a big drum
> hammering a nail
> chopping wood
> swatting at a mosquito
> swinging a bat

Observation and Evaluation: Does the child demonstrate striking at the air only? Does the child correctly execute a strike? Can the child identify with the imagery used?

Adding Equipment: Some children may find it helpful to actually practice striking an object. Balloons are perfect for this purpose because their bright colors make them easy to track visually and they are easy to keep in the air! (*Note:* Because of the potential choking hazard, children should never be allowed to handle deflated balloons.)

Curriculum Connectors: The self-expression inherent with pretending falls under the heading of *social studies*. You can add *music* and *language arts* to the mix by singing the following lyrics to the tune of "Farmer in the Dell:"

Watch me strike the air.
Now watch me strike again.
I can strike with first one arm
And then the other one.

Let's Roll

A log roll is generally defined as a movement made by a body that is supine (face up) or prone (face down) and fully extended, with the arms stretched overhead. Introduce the children to this type of roll, and then ask them to try it. (*Note:* If you work with a large number of children, it might be best to perform this at first with small groups.)

Extending the Activity: Mastering this skill will take lots of practice. Challenge children to perform it in both directions, both slowly and quickly. Can they make their bodies stay as straight as logs—or pencils?

Observation and Evaluation: Is the child able to assume a straight body position, fully extended and with arms stretched overhead? Can the child keep the body straight while rolling? Can the child roll in both directions?

Adding Equipment: Using a pencil to demonstrate how this roll should look can definitely help!

Curriculum Connectors: *Language arts* are included here because directionality is essential to emergent literacy, and *slowly* and *quickly* are opposites. Sing the following, to the tune of "Where Is Thumbkin?," to add more language arts and also *music* to the experience:

Watch me rolling,
Watch me rolling.
Here I go, here I go.
Watch me rolling quickly,
Watch me rolling quickly.
Now nice and slow,
Nice and slow.

The Bumblebee

 "The Bumblebee" (Length 1:07)—CD Track 12

This song focuses on quick movement, with the children pretending to be bumblebees "buzzing" around the room. These are the lyrics:

The bumblebee goes buzz, buzz, buzz,
From one flower to the next.
The bumblebee goes buzz, buzz, buzz,
That is what a bumblebee does!
So buzz, buzz, buzz like a bumblebee.
Buzzing here, everywhere.
Yes, buzz, buzz, buzz like a bumblebee.
You'll have fun, I guarantee!

Extending the Activity: Encourage children to "buzz" in straight, curving, and zigzag pathways; high in the air and nearer to the floor; and stopping occasionally to "land on a flower."

Observation and Evaluation: Does the child remain in control while moving quickly? Can the child vary the movement as suggested?

Curriculum Connectors: Consideration of an insect and its movement falls under the heading of *science*, while the song provides experience with both *language arts* and *music*.

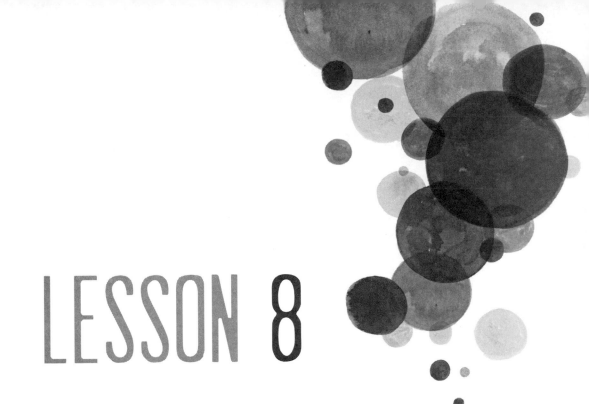

LESSON 8

See My Feet

Talk to the children about all the different things their feet help them do, and then ask them to show you how they move when they do the following things. Possibilities include these:

walking	climbing stairs
running	kicking a ball
skating	stamping
jumping	dancing

Extending the Activity: Ask the children to suggest other things their feet help them do. Possibilities include tiptoeing, hiking, skiing, and bouncing. Challenge them to demonstrate.

Observation and Evaluation: Does the child understand the concept involved and the various roles performed by the feet? Does the child properly execute the skills being demonstrated?

Adding Equipment: *Dribbling* is a manipulative skill performed in such activities as soccer. Because a ball is too dynamic, and therefore difficult to manage, young children can begin practicing this skill with beanbags. Simply invite them to experiment by pushing the beanbag around the floor with their feet.

Curriculum Connectors: Exploration of the functions of a particular body part constitutes *science* for young children.

Let's Push and Pull

Discuss pushing and pulling with the children, particularly the aspect of *resistance* that is part of both of these skills. What are some things that have to be pushed or pulled? Show children some classroom toys that can be pushed and pulled, like a wagon, push or pull toys, a child-sized grocery cart, and so on. Then, emphasizing that these exercises are imaginary and must be performed without touching each other, ask the children to push, and then pull, in the following ways:

- with both hands
- with one hand and then the other, alternately
- forward; downward; upward; sideways
- very slowly; quickly
- strong and hard; lightly (against less resistance)

Extending the Activity: Add imagery to the activity by asking the children to pretend to do these things:

- push a swing at the playground
- pull a kite through the air
- push heavy furniture
- pull a heavy anchor out of the water
- push a balloon into the air
- pull a wagon or a sled
- push a car stuck in mud or snow
- push a lawn mower
- pull a balloon down from the sky
- push a grocery cart

Observation and Evaluation: Does the child demonstrate knowledge of a marked difference between pushing and pulling? Does the child understand the concept of resistance (for example, some things are harder to push or pull than others)?

Adding Equipment: It may help to have actual items of various weights for the children to experiment with. Possibilities include a balloon, wagon, chair, and pull toy.

Curriculum Connectors: Resistance is a concept falling under the heading of *science*.

Marching Band

● ●

♪ **"Marching Band" (Length 1:46)—CD Track 13**

Children love to march and pretend that they are in a parade. Play this song and encourage your toddlers to march both in place and around the room. Don't worry if some children do not march right on the beat—it is early yet!

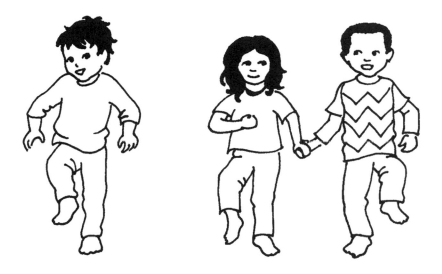

Extending the Activity: If possible, show children pictures of a marching band, discussing the different instruments being played. Then play the song again, challenging children to march while pretending to play the instrument of their choice. (*Note:* Children will most likely be familiar with playing drums but may require a demonstration from you when other instruments are involved. Also, some children may not yet be ready to play and march at the same time; they will either march without "playing an instrument" or will stand still while pretending to play the instrument.)

Observation and Evaluation: Does the child march with good posture and limbs in opposition? Is the child able to march on the beat? Can the child march and "play an instrument" at the same time?

Adding Equipment: Adding real rhythm band instruments to the activity will certainly make it noisier, but it will also make it more fun for your toddlers!

Curriculum Connectors: A march is a style of *music*. You might also choose to discuss certain holidays during which parades are held to incorporate *social studies*.

Moving Backward

So far you have not had the children focus exclusively on moving in a backward direction. However, by now they will have acquired a respect for movement and for personal space, and they should be ready for this activity.

Ask the children to move backward in the following ways:

- walking
- jumping
- with little (big) steps
- on hands and feet (hands and knees; for example, creeping)
- crawling (for example, on the tummy)

Extending the Activity: Perform Follow the Leader exclusively in a backward direction, each time using more challenging movements and movement elements, varying their pathways, levels, speed, and force.

Curriculum Connectors: Direction is a spatial concept relevant to *art*, *mathematics*, and *language arts*.

LESSON 9

See My Face

Sit with the children and explain how they are going to discover the many different things they can do and say with just their faces alone. Then present the following challenges to them. (*Note:* Because this is exploration, or divergent problem solving, you should only demonstrate if the children are not sure how to respond. Otherwise, they will imitate you instead of finding their own "solutions.")

- Let me see a smile; a frown.
- Make a "growling" face.
- Close your eyes really tight; open them wide.
- Wiggle your nose the way a bunny rabbit does.
- Close your mouth tightly; open it wide like a tunnel.
- Can you make your mouth move from side to side?
- Pucker up, as if you have just sucked on a sour lemon.
- Blink your eyes open and shut like a light going on and off.
- Lick your lips, as if you have just seen something yummy to eat.
- Show me a surprised face!
- Show me an angry face.
- Can you show me a really sad, about-to-cry face?
- Show me a happy face!

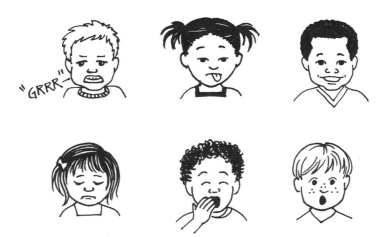

Extending the Activity: Act out the following poem, first discussing some of the terms that may be unfamiliar to the children (for example, *role* means "job"). When you come to the last verse, ask the children to cover their faces with their hands and, on the final line, disclose their "very own" faces, the faces they would most like you to see, or the funniest ones they can make.

A face has many roles in life,
I guess you know that's true.
It smiles and frowns and even cries
When you are feeling blue.
A face can show you're angry;
A face can show you're glad.
A face can pout and sulk and whine
When you are feeling bad.

A face can show that you're tired
With yawns or drooping eyes.
A face can even show delight
When someone yells "Surprise!"
A face has many roles in life,
But most unique by far—
'Cause yours belongs to only you,
I can tell who you are!

Observation and Evaluation: Does the child identify with the images and emotions involved? Does the child participate?

Curriculum Connectors: Self-expression is central to early *social studies* for young children; body-part identification and exploration constitute *science*. Using the poem adds *language arts* to the mix.

The Tightrope

● ●

♪ "Circus Medley" (Length 3:55)—CD Track 14

For this activity you will need tightropes, whether imaginary or created by masking tape, yarn, or rope on the floor. Most toddlers will find a visible tightrope much easier. You will want to make more than one or two available, however, so the children do not have to wait long for a turn.

After presenting the tightropes, ask the children to pretend they are tightrope walkers in the circus, balancing high above the crowd. This may require some discussion or pictures, and you might want to remind them that there is a net below! Also, like real tightrope walkers, they should extend their arms to the sides to provide additional balance. Accompany this activity with "Circus Medley" to provide the appropriate atmosphere.

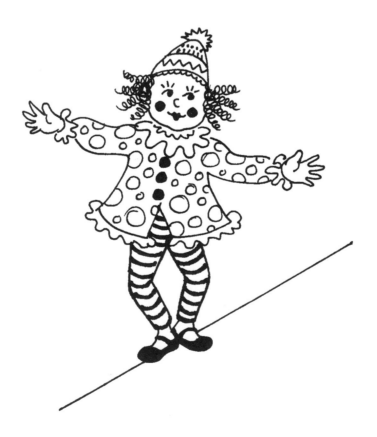

Extending the Activity: Once the children have demonstrated an ability to move forward across the "tightrope," invite them to try moving sideways. Can they try it moving backward?

Observation and Evaluation: Does the child place arms out to sides and one foot in front of the other while attempting to "walk the tightrope"? Can the child maintain balance while moving in forward, sideways, and backward directions?

Adding Equipment: The tightrope can be just one part of an obstacle course set up indoors or outdoors. Other components might include tunnels, large cardboard boxes, mats, foam crawl-through shapes, low balance beams, and plastic hoops.

Curriculum Connectors: Balance is a concept falling under the heading of *science*, while any discussion of circus performer as occupation constitutes *social studies*. Using "Circus Medley" provides experience with *music*.

Follow the Leader

Rather than leading the children in a line, move about the room so all the children can see you, using different forms of locomotion, which your children must imitate. Possibilities include walking or running in these ways:

- with big (small) steps
- lightly; heavily
- in slow motion; quickly
- with the body in different shapes, arms out to sides, body as small or large as possible, and so on

Extending the Activity: Each time you perform this activity, make your movements more challenging. Move in straight, curving, and zigzag pathways; in forward, sideways, and backward directions; at low, middle, and high levels; adding stops and starts to the movement.

Observation and Evaluation: Is the child able to physically replicate what the eyes are seeing? In what way(s) is the child unable to respond?

Adding Equipment: To make the activity even more challenging, you can include *prop* movement, which the children must also replicate. Possible props are scarves, ribbon sticks, or rhythm band instruments.

Curriculum Connectors: Being able to physically replicate what the eyes see is central to *art* and to reading and writing (*language arts*). Using rhythm band instruments will offer experience with elements of *music*.

Marching Slow/Marching Fast

♪ **"Marching Slow/Marching Fast" (Length 1:31)—CD Track 15**

"Marching Slow/Marching Fast" offers two different marching tempos, requiring more bodily control from the children. For this lesson, simply play the tape and ask the children to march accordingly. The form of the song is AB, with A being the slow march and B the fast march.

Extending the Activity: As with "Marching Band" (page 81), you can invite children to imagine they are also playing an instrument typically found in a marching band. Other possibilities include carrying a flag or banner or twirling a baton.

Observation and Evaluation: Does the child march with good posture and limbs in opposition? Does the child demonstrate an awareness of the difference in tempos? Is the child able to move appropriately in response to both the slow and fast tempos?

Adding Equipment: Rhythm band instruments can enhance the experience. Chiffon scarves and streamers can be used to represent flags.

Curriculum Connectors: A march is a style of *music*, while the element of time is relevant to *mathematics*. Again, you can include *social studies* by discussing holidays that are typically celebrated with parades.

LESSON 10

Mirror Game

· ·

As part of their development, children must continue to learn to physically imitate what they experience visually. This game, which is similar to Simon Says, gives them the opportunity to do just that.

Standing where all of the children can easily see you, explain that they should pretend to be your reflection in the mirror, imitating your every move. If possible, demonstrate this in front of a large mirror, or talk to them about times they have looked at themselves in a mirror. You then move parts of your body in various ways (for example, raising and lowering an arm; tilting your head), slowly and without verbal instruction; and the children do likewise.

Extending the Activity: To make this game more challenging, pick up—and frequently change—the pace of your movements. Also, make subtler movements—with smaller body parts. For example, you might raise your eyebrows or wiggle your fingers with your arms by your sides. This requires that the children really pay attention!

Observation and Evaluation: Is the child able to physically replicate what the eyes are seeing? Does the child have control over the body parts involved?

Adding Equipment: You can add something brightly colored—such as chiffon scarves—to this activity to make your hand and arm movements easier to track visually. The children, who are also holding scarves, should move their arms in the same directions and shapes as yours.

Curriculum Connectors: Physically imitating what is being experienced visually is essential to *language arts* and is also a central component of *art*, as are the concepts of space and shape. The concept of a mirror reflection is relative to *science*.

Let's Lift

Pretending to lift objects will be more challenging for toddlers than such activities as pulling, pushing, or striking. However, with enough verbalization concerning the size, weight, and shape of these imaginary objects, even young children (toddlers) should experience some success.

Ask the children to pretend to lift such diverse things as these:

balloon   big bag of groceries

cement block   shovel full of snow

baby from a crib   handkerchief

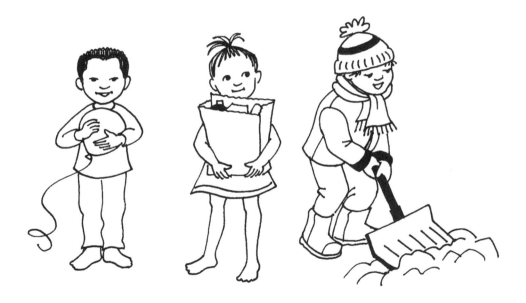

Extending the Activity: Body parts can be lifted too. Challenge the children to demonstrate how they can lift their arms, legs, knees, chin, shoulders, elbows, toes, and fingers!

Observation and Evaluation: Does the child understand the difference between light and heavy lifting? Is the child able to respond to the imagery used? Is the child able to identify and lift the designated body parts?

Adding Equipment: It may help to first practice lifting real objects of varying weights and sizes and ask the children to think about the amount of effort required in lifting each object. Possible objects include a balloon, chair, chiffon scarf, beach ball, blocks, canned vegetables or fruit, and books.

Curriculum Connectors: Weight and size are relative to *mathematics*. The amount of effort required to lift varying weights and sizes is applicable to *science*, as is body-part identification.

Moving Like the Animals

Talk about the characteristics of the following animals, showing pictures if you can, and then ask the children to show you how they would move if they were one of these animals:

chicken	rabbit
monkey	kangaroo
racehorse	bird
huge, heavy elephant	lion or tiger
dog	turtle

Extending the Activity: Once the children have demonstrated that they can move like different animals, challenge them to vary their pathways (straight, curving, and zigzag) and levels. For example, if they have been depicting a chicken while moving at a middle level, encourage them to show you how a chicken would move closer to the floor. How would a horse, dog, or elephant move in a circle?

Observation and Evaluation: Does the child distinguish among these animals (for example, demonstrate different kinds of movement)? Can the child demonstrate the appropriate movements?

Curriculum Connectors: Consideration of a variety of animals and their movements constitutes *science*.

Slow-Motion Moving

♪ **"Slow-Motion Moving" (Length 1:21)—CD Track 16**

As this song plays, ask the children to portray different animals or objects that move very slowly. Remember—moving very slowly does not come naturally to young children, but that doesn't mean you can't ask them to try!

Some suggested images follow. However, if you find these movements are too advanced for your group, you can simply ask the children to show you how slowly they can move.

- a turtle crawling
- a candle (or ice cube) melting
- a seed growing
- a flower opening
- a baby learning to walk

Extending the Activity: Talk to the children about wind-up toys, explaining that they move quickly at first but gradually wind down, getting slower and slower. Then "wind them up" (it's fun if each child can be wound up individually), and ask the children to move like a toy. You may have to remind them to gradually slow their movements.

Observation and Evaluation: Does the child exhibit the necessary control to move slowly? Can the child relate to the imagery used? Does the child demonstrate an ability to gradually slow down?

Adding Equipment: For the purposes of the alternate activity, demonstrating with an actual wind-up toy can definitely help.

Curriculum Connectors: Tempo is an element of *music*; time is related to *mathematics*.

LESSON 11

Simon Says

. . . .

This is an excellent body-parts activity, as it is challenging yet familiar to most children. I propose one major change, though: do it without the elimination process. In the traditional game, the children who need to participate the most are usually the first to be eliminated. Besides, elimination goes against the grain of a success-oriented philosophy! Initially, you should say "Simon says" before each of the following challenges. (*Note:* If your children do not understand the concept of your pretending to be someone called "Simon," have a favorite stuffed animal state the commands, using the animal's name in place of "Simon.")

Raise your arms.

Touch your head.

Stand up tall.

Touch your shoulders.

Pucker up your mouth.

Stand on one foot.

Place your hands on your hips.

Bend and touch your knees.

Close (then open) your eyes.

Reach for the sky.

Give yourself a hug!

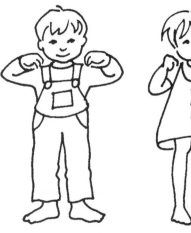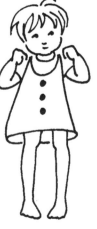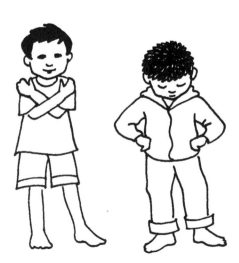

Extending the Activity: To make the activity more challenging—and to emphasize listening skills—play the game the traditional way, sometimes saying "Simon says" and sometimes not saying it. However, place the children in two separate circles or lines first. Then, instead of being eliminated, children who move without Simon's permission can simply change groups or lines, allowing for constant participation and more chances to succeed!

Observation and Evaluation: Can the child identify all body parts? Does the child exhibit the necessary listening skills?

Curriculum Connectors: Listening skills are components of both *language arts* and *music*. Body-part identification falls under the heading of *science* for young children.

Let's Balance

Balance, of course, is a necessary skill for everyone. With the following challenges, children become familiar with the concept of balance at a low level. Depending on the ages of your children, probably not everyone will succeed with these exercises, but it is fun to try them anyway!

Ask the children to balance in these ways:

on hands and knees only
on two hands and one knee
on one hand and one knee
on bottom only
on tummy only

Next, invite the children to experiment with a variety of balances at a high level. Ask them to try balancing in these ways:

on tiptoe
on one foot (flat), then the other
with arms out to sides (and flat-footed), leaning forward, backward, and to either
    side as far as possible

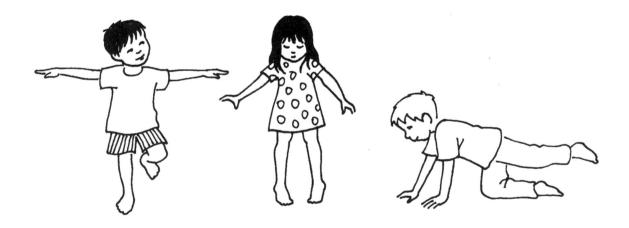

Extending the Activity: Some of the following challenges are more difficult than others (some even for adults!), but they are all fun to try. Ask your toddlers to try balancing in the following ways:

> on tiptoe ("How long can you stay up there?")
> on tiptoe with knees bent ("How low can you go?")
> either on tiptoe or standing on one foot, with arms extended to sides and upper
>   body leaning in different directions
> on one foot on tiptoe

Observation and Evaluation: Does the child understand the concept of balance? In what ways is the child able to balance? In what ways is the child unable to balance?

Curriculum Connectors: Balance is a concept falling under the heading of *science*, as is the recognition of body parts. The concept of levels in space is a component of *art*. The one-to-one correspondence involving body parts means *mathematics* is also involved.

Let's Tiptoe

Generally speaking, you can expect your toddlers to take about four steps on tiptoe by the time they reach twenty-seven months. Give walking on tiptoe a try here, and see what happens!

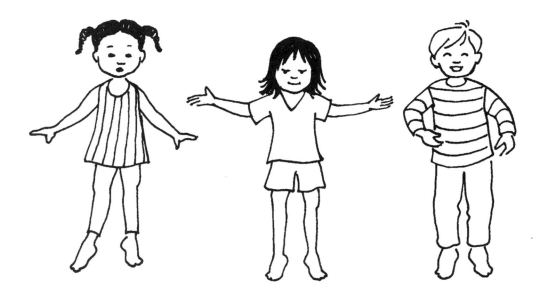

Extending the Activity: Invite the children to imagine they are cats sneaking up on something. What is it about the way cats use their paws that enable them to move so quietly?

Observation and Evaluation: Does the child move on the balls of the feet only? Is the child able to maintain balance while tiptoeing?

Adding Equipment: Provide a "tightrope" once again, in the form of a rope or masking tape on the floor, and ask the children to try tiptoeing from one end to the other.

Curriculum Connectors: Pretending to be a cat constitutes *science*, as does experimenting with balance.

The Tiptoe Song

 "The Tiptoe Song" (Length 1:04)—CD Track 17

Tiptoeing is used here specifically as a method of exploring the movement element of force. For this activity, the children simply tiptoe along with the song. The lyrics are:

Can you tiptoe
Very quietly?
Can you tiptoe
Gently as can be?
Softly, softly,
Lightly do you go.
Softly, softly,
That's how you tiptoe!
Sh-h-h-h!

Extending the Activity: Once children have mastered tiptoeing in a forward direction, challenge them to try it in sideways and backward directions. Suggest they try it both slowly and quickly, in different pathways and at different levels.

Observation and Evaluation: Is the child moving *lightly*? Does the child understand the concept of moving lightly?

Curriculum Connectors: Tiptoeing requires moving lightly, and *light* and *heavy* are quantitative concepts falling under *mathematics*, as well as opposites (*language arts*). Of course, the song involves both language arts and *music* (the musical element of volume is explored).

LESSON 12

The Body Song

. . . .

♪ "The Body Song" (Length 2:11)—CD Track 18

Read each line of the following poem as slowly as necessary to allow the children ample time to respond—but not enough time to let boredom overtake those who respond more quickly.

Show me you can touch your toes,
Then bring your hand up to your nose.
Put a smile upon your face,
Do it all in your own space!
Bring your elbows to your knees,
Then shake all over, if you please.
Straighten up with hands on hips.
Can you pucker up those lips?

Touch your ankle with your hand.
Upon one foot can you now stand?
Wiggle fingers in the air.
Shake your hips now, if you dare.
Close your eyes, then open quick.
Around your lips let your tongue lick.
With your shoulders you can shrug.
Give yourself a great big hug!

Extending the Activity: When the children are ready, do the activity musically. The song is the same as the poem, only set to music and with a chorus. To the words of the chorus, they should open and close their arms (twice) on the first and third lines, and shrug on the second line. The fourth line is self-explanatory!

The chorus is as follows:

The body, the body;
What parts do you know?
The body, your body;
Touch it high and low!

Observation and Evaluation: Is the child able to identify all body parts? Does the child respond appropriately to the challenges presented in the poem (song)?

Curriculum Connectors: These activities provide children experiences with body-part identification (*science*), *language arts*, and *music*. Also, the concepts of high and low are part of both *art* and *mathematics*.

Shake, Wiggle, and Vibrate

. . . .

Talk about the meaning of these words—and about their images—with the children. How do shaking, wiggling, and vibrating differ from each other? Then ask your toddlers to show you they can move in the following ways. Demonstrate only if necessary:

> move like a snake
> look like soup sloshing in a bowl
> shake and vibrate like a baby's rattle
> wiggle like you are being tickled
> look like a leaf in the wind
> shake as though very, very cold
> vibrate like a battery-powered toothbrush

Extending the Activity: Challenge the children to shake, wiggle, or vibrate individual body parts, like the head, a hand, arm, or foot. Most likely, the whole body will shake, wiggle, and vibrate along with the individual part, but experimenting with it will be fun anyway!

Observation and Evaluation: Can the child identify with the imagery used? Does the child demonstrate understanding of the differences among shaking, wiggling, and vibrating?

Adding Equipment: Using a maraca or a rain stick can help the children *hear* the differences among shaking, wiggling, and vibrating and may especially help with the concept of vibration.

Curriculum Connectors: Shaking, wiggling, and vibrating all require different amounts of muscle tension, qualifying these activities as *science*.

Let's Jump Again

More opportunity to practice jumping! Ask the children to jump in these ways:

forward

backward

to the side (the other side)

in a circle

Now repeat those activities, asking the children to try them again with their arms in a variety of positions so they get used to letting their feet and legs do the work. Ask them to jump in these ways:

arms folded across chest

arms out to sides

hands on hips

hands clasped behind the back

Extending the Activity: Emphasizing height, invite your toddlers to try jumping in these ways:

light (heavy) jumps

jumping like bouncing balls—some high, some low

jumping and turning

jumping as though reaching for something high

Observation and Evaluation: Does the child use the feet and legs to push off the floor? Does the child land toe-ball-heel, with knees bent?

Adding Equipment: Providing something for children to jump *over* can often help with both the concept and practice of jumping—and makes it more fun! Start with jump ropes or hoops lying flat on the floor and then move on to something with a bit of height, like small plastic cones.

Curriculum Connectors: Directions and positional concepts like high, low, and over are part of both *mathematics* and *art*.

Moving Softly/Moving Loudly

♪ **"Moving Softly/Moving Loudly" (Length 1:30)—CD Track 19**

Suggest that the children move in ways requiring less force during the soft parts of this song and in more forceful ways during the louder parts. Suggestions include these:

Soft	Loud
moving arms gently	moving arms strongly
patting softly	pounding fists in air
swaying gently	rocking forcefully

Extending the Activity: The following images alternate between those requiring less force and muscle tension and those requiring more. Talk about the following images, and then ask the children to move like each of these things:

- a feather floating through the air
- a robot
- a floppy rag doll
- a tin soldier
- a butterfly
- an angry person
- a cat sneaking up on something

Also, you may have to model for the children during early experiences with "Moving Softly/Moving Loudly." However, during later explorations, encourage your toddlers to find their own ways of moving to the soft and loud music.

Observation and Evaluation: Does the child seem to differentiate between soft and loud music? Does the child demonstrate a difference between moving lightly and moving strongly?

Curriculum Connectors: The concepts of force and muscle tension are linked to *science*. The concept of volume (*music*) is also being explored with the song.

LESSON 13

Body-Part Balance

Here the children are asked to place their weight only on the body part or parts you have indicated. You then count to five, challenging the children to hold as still as possible while balancing on these parts.

Ask them to balance on the following parts only:

hands and knees

hands and feet

knees and elbows

back

one (then the other) side of the body

tummy

bottom

knees

Extending the Activity: A more challenging activity is to ask the children to shift their weight smoothly from one position to the next, using the list above. For example, the children will first be balancing on their hands and knees. You will then challenge them to shift smoothly onto their hands and feet, and so on. This exercise may require demonstration and/or physical assistance in some cases. Physiologically, because of the weight of the head, this activity is going to be difficult; but it is okay if the children lose their balance—it's fun!

Observation and Evaluation: Does the child properly identify body parts? Is the child able to achieve and maintain balance? Does the child understand the concept of shifting weight, and is the child able to perform this?

Curriculum Connectors: Balance, the shifting of weight, and body-part identification all fall under the heading of *science*. Counting constitutes simple *mathematics*.

High and Low

 "High and Low" (Length 1:13)—CD Track 20

With the children sitting, start this song. Then, as the music gradually gets higher and higher, have the children raise their arms. (You should do it too.) Then have the children lower their arms as the music descends. Note that a resting space is provided before the ascent begins again.

The pattern is:

8 counts up; 8 counts down
8 counts up; 8 counts down
8-count rest

4 counts up; 4 counts down
4 counts up; 4 counts down
8-count rest

2 counts up; 2 counts down; repeat twice
8-count rest

8 counts up; 4 counts down
4 counts up; 4 counts down
8-count rest

2 counts up; 8 counts down; repeat
2 counts up

Extending the Activity: The next step is to begin the song as the children are crouching low. Then, as the music gradually gets higher and higher, so do the children. Next they descend with the music. Eventually the children should be able to do this without you modeling, letting only the sound of the music dictate their movements.

Observation and Evaluation: Is the child imitating the modeled movements? Does the child appear to understand/hear the concept of ascending and descending notes?

Adding Equipment: Holding a brightly colored chiffon scarf in each hand can make the activity more visually appealing and may therefore contribute to a greater understanding of *ascending* and *descending*.

Curriculum Connectors: This song explores the concept of pitch in *music*. *Up* and *down* are positional concepts that are important to both *mathematics* and *art*, and listening skills are also essential to *language arts*.

Let's Crawl

Brain research has pointed to the importance of cross-lateral movement in the development of reading and writing skills, so this type of movement is something young children can never get too much of. Although crawling is the child's earliest form of locomotor movement, it is seldom practiced once the child is able to travel on foot. Crawling involves lying on the stomach, with head and shoulders raised off the floor and the weight of the upper torso supported by the elbows. Locomotion involves moving the elbows and hips.

Talk to the children about worms, snakes, and seals and how they move, providing pictures if possible. Then invite your toddlers to pretend to be each of these creatures.

Extending the Activity: Demonstrate homolateral crawling for the children, in which the arm and leg on the same side of the body move simultaneously. Then invite the children to try it themselves!

Observation and Evaluation: Does the child correctly execute the crawl? Is the child able to perform homolateral, as well as cross-lateral, movement?

Adding Equipment: Providing tunnels for the children to crawl through can help motivate them to keep practicing this basic skill.

Curriculum Connectors: Practicing moving the way various creatures move falls under the heading of *science*. Cross-lateral movement is essential to the *language arts* skills of reading and writing.

Robots and Astronauts

🎵 **"Robots and Astronauts" (Length 1:46)—CD Track 21**

This song gives children opportunities to experience the elements of force and flow. The robots section (A) requires more force and is an example of *bound flow* (punctuated, halting). The astronauts section (B) requires less force and is an example of *free flow* (uninterrupted).

Play the song, the form of which is AB. Ask the children to pretend to be robots during part A, then ask them to pretend they are astronauts, floating weightlessly in outer space, during part B.

Extending the Activity: What other images come to mind during this song? After pretending to be robots and astronauts, the children could perhaps pretend to be tin soldiers and eagles soaring.

Observation and Evaluation: Does the child use more muscle tension and move in a stilted manner during the A section? Does the child use less muscle tension and move in a smooth manner during the B section? Is the child able to transition from one type of movement to the other?

Adding Equipment: To further explore the movement element of *flow*, which is probably the most abstract for young children, play a game of Traffic Lights. This activity requires three pieces of paper (or cardboard or objects) in the colors red, green, and yellow. Talk to the children about traffic lights and what they mean to drivers and pedestrians. Then explain that you are going to hold up different colors (the same colors as traffic lights) that will tell them how to move. (They can pretend to be driving cars if they like.) When the children see green, they should walk around; red means stop; and yellow means walk in place.

Curriculum Connectors: The concept of muscle tension falls under the heading of *science*. The song explores the concepts of *staccato* (the robot sound) and *legato* (the astronaut sound) in *music*. The traffic-lights activity brings in *social studies*.

LESSON 14

Traveling Body Parts

This activity gives the children additional practice with body parts, as well as providing them with a better idea of the range of their personal space. (*Note:* Remind the children, if necessary, that their personal space is the area surrounding the body, like a giant bubble.)

Ask your toddlers to sit with their hands in their laps. Then instruct them to make one hand travel far away from the other, without moving their bodies from their spots. Next, ask the children to leave the first hand where it is and move the other hand to meet it. Can the first hand then travel far away again, but in a different direction?

Extending the Activity: Once the children get the hang of this, you can try the same activity with legs, elbows, wrists, knees, or feet.

Observation and Evaluation: Does the child readily identify body parts? Does the child demonstrate an understanding of personal space? Does the child understand the concepts of *far* and *near*?

Adding Equipment: Using stretch bands (available from movement education suppliers) or stretchy fabric can help children see the amount of space involved as they move their body parts away from and nearer to each other.

Curriculum Connectors: Personal space and the concepts of far and near are part of both *art* and *mathematics*. Body-part identification is part of *science*.

In My Space

 "In My Space" (Length 2:42)—CD Track 22

This song serves as a review of the many activities the children have learned to do in their own spaces. Ask the children to act out the lines accordingly.

Here are the lyrics:

See me stretch
And see me bend.
See me turn around.
Now see me turn the other way,
All without a sound!
See me push
Into the air.
Now just watch me pull.
I can even pretend to lift.
Isn't it wonderful?

See me sway
From side to side.
Now I'm going to shake.
See me shake myself to the floor.
It's time to take a break!
Chorus: *I can stay in just one spot*
And do so many things.
It's true that I can do a lot
Do you want to see?

Extending the Activity: Challenge children to show you how many ways they can find to stretch, bend, turn, push, pull, lift, sway, and shake. Or, if the concept of *how many* is still too difficult for them, limit the challenge to finding two or three different ways.

Observation and Evaluation: Is the child able to perform all of the nonlocomotor skills involved?

Curriculum Connectors: In addition to *music* and *language arts*, this song offers experience with personal space, a concept relevant to both *art* and *mathematics*.

Follow the Leader

In the reprise of this activity, lead the children throughout the room in the traditional manner, being sure to incorporate all of the locomotor skills they have so far experienced and practiced. Also, include a variety of body shapes, tempos, directions, levels, pathways, stops and starts, and different amounts of force.

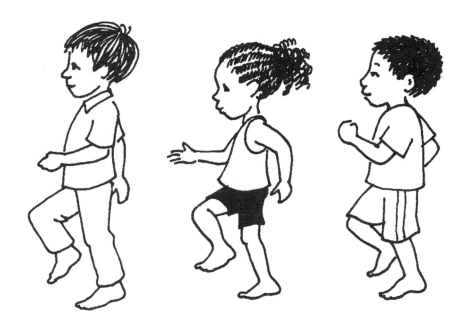

Extending the Activity: Practice those locomotor skills and movement elements with which the children may have had some difficulty. Begin to introduce such new locomotor skills as *leaping* and *hopping*.

Observation and Evaluation: Is the child able to physically replicate what the eyes are seeing? Which movement skills and elements is the child having trouble with?

Curriculum Connectors: The ability to physically replicate what the eyes are seeing is central to *art* and *language arts*. By varying the speed, force, direction, and so on of the movement, you are also incorporating elements of *mathematics* and *science*.

Common Meters

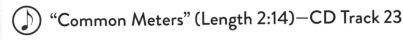

♪ "Common Meters" (Length 2:14)—CD Track 23

This song is in four parts, performed in the common meters of 2/4, 3/4, 4/4, and 6/8. It is not important that the children understand the technical differences among them, however. What is important is that the children be exposed to various meters and that they have the opportunity to experience them physically. So play the song and ask the children to move in the following ways:

> 2/4: clapping 1-2; stamping 1-2; marching; jumping
> 3/4: swaying; swinging arms; clapping 1-2-3
> 4/4: clapping 1-2-3-4; running; nodding; conducting an orchestra
> 6/8: marching; clapping 1-2; moving head side to side; rocking

Extending the Activity: Allow the children to find their own ways of moving to the four different parts of the song.

Observation and Evaluation: Does the child seem to differentiate among the four meters by moving in varying ways?

Adding Equipment: Provide each child with a rhythm instrument with which to experiment as the music is playing.

Curriculum Connectors: The concept of meter is one of the elements of *music* to which children should definitely be exposed. Counting is part of *mathematics*.

References

AAHPERD (American Alliance for Health, Physical Education, Recreation and Dance). 2009. *Active Start: A Statement of Physical Activity Guidelines for Children from Birth to Age 5*. 2nd ed. Reston, VA: AAHPERD.

Amabile, Teresa M. 1992. *Growing Up Creative: Nurturing a Lifetime of Creativity*. 2nd ed. Buffalo, NY: The Creative Education Foundation Press.

Bar-Or, Oded, John Foreyt, Claude Bouchard, Kelly D. Brownell, William H. Dietz, Eric Ravussin, Arline D. Salbe, Sandy Schwenger, Sachico St. Jeor, and Benjamin Torun. 1998. "Physical Activity, Genetic, and Nutritional Considerations in Childhood Weight Management." *Medicine and Science in Sports and Exercise* 30 (1): 2–10.

Carson, Linda M. 2001. "The 'I Am Learning' Curriculum: Developing a Movement Awareness in Young Children." *Teaching Elementary Physical Education* 12 (5): 9–13. Choosykids.com/CK2resources/eventhost/Day%202 /Body%20Language/The%201%20am%20Moving%20Curriculum.pdf.

CDC (Centers for Disease Control and Prevention). 2008. "Preventing Diabetes and Its Complications." http://www.cdc.gov/nccdphp/publications/fact sheets/prevention/pdf/diabetes.pdf.

Frostig, Marianne. 1970. *Movement Education: Theory and Practice*. Chicago: Follett Education Corporation.

Gallahue, David L., and Frances Cleland Donnelly. 2003. *Developmental Physical Education for All Children*. 4th ed. Champaign, IL: Human Kinetics.

Halsey, Elizabeth, and Lorena Porter. 1970. "Movement Exploration." In *Selected Readings in Movement Education*, edited by Robert T. Sweeney, 71–77. Reading, MA: Addison-Wesley Publishing Company.

Hannaford, Carla. 2005. *Smart Moves: Why Learning Is Not All in Your Head*. 2nd ed. Salt Lake City, UT: Great River Books.

H'Doubler, Margaret Newell. 1925. *The Dance and Its Place in Education*. New York: Harcourt, Brace, and Company.

Kaur, Harsohena, Won S. Choi, Matthew S. Mayo, and Kari Jo Harris. 2003. "Duration of Television Watching Is Associated with Body Mass Index." *Journal of Pediatrics* 143 (4): 506–11. doi:10.1067/S0022-3476(03)00418-9.

Lewin, Tamar. 2010. "If Your Kids Are Awake, They're Probably Online." *New York Times*, January 20. http://www.nytimes.com/2010/01/20/education/20wired .html.

Mayesky, Mary. 2009. *Creative Activities for Young Children.* 9th ed. Clifton Park, NY: Delmar.

McDonough, Patricia. 2009. "Television and Beyond a Kid's Eye View." http:// www.nielsen.com/us/en/newswire/2009/television-and-beyond-a-kids-eye -view.html.

Mosston, Muska, and Sara Ashworth. 1990. *The Spectrum of Teaching Styles: From Command to Discovery.* New York: Longman.

NAEYC (National Association for the Education of Young Children). 2009a. *Developmentally Appropriate Practice in Early Childhood Programs Serving Children from Birth through Age 8.* Position statement. Washington, DC: NAEYC. www.naeyc.org/files/naeyc/file/positions/PSDAP.pdf.

———. 2009b. *NAEYC Standards for Early Childhood Professional Preparation Programs.* Position statement. Washington, DC: NAEYC. http://www.naeyc .org/files/naeyc/file/positions/ProfPrepStandards09.pdf.

NIEER (National Institute for Early Education Research). 2010. "Preschool's Role in Fighting Childhood Obesity." *Preschool Matters* 8 (1): 12. http://nieer .org/sites/nieer/files/81.pdf.

Pate, Russell R., Kerry McIver, Marsha Dowda, William H. Brown, and Cheryl Addy. 2008. "Directly Observed Physical Activity Levels in Preschool Children." *Journal of School Health* 78 (8): 438–44. doi:10.1111/j.1746-1561.2008.00327.x.

Samuelson, Emily. 1981. "Group Development and Socialization through Movement." In *Readings: Developing Arts Programs for Handicapped Students*, edited by Lola H. Kearns, Mary Taylor Ditson, and Bernice Gottschalk Roehner, 53–54. Harrisburg, PA: Arts in Special Education Project of Pennsylvania.

Science Daily. 2010. "Obese Children Show Signs of Heart Disease Typically Seen in Middle-Aged Adults, Researcher Says." http://www.sciencedaily.com /releases/2010/10/101025005835.htm.

Additional Resources

Sources for Ordering Musical Instruments

Childcraft

www.childcrafteducation.com

888-388-3224

Constructive Playthings

www.constructiveplaythings.com

800-448-1412

Lakeshore

www.lakeshorelearning.com

800-428-4414

MMB Music

www.mmbmusic.com

314-531-9635

Music in Motion

www.musicmotion.com

800-807-3520

Rhythm Band Instruments

www.rhythmband.com

800-424-4724

Sources for Ordering Equipment and Props

FlagHouse
www.flaghouse.com
800-793-7900

Kaplan Early Learning Company
www.kaplanco.com
800-334-2014

Lakeshore Learning
www.lakeshorelearning.com
800-428-4414

Play with a Purpose
www.pwaponline.com
888-330-1826

US Games
www.usgames.com
800-327-0484

About the Author

Rae Pica is an internationally recognized education consultant specializing in early childhood physical activity. Known for her lively and informative presentations and keynote speeches, she has also consulted for such groups as the *Sesame Street* Research Department, the Head Start Bureau, the Centers for Disease Control and Prevention, the President's Council on Physical Fitness and Sports, Nickelodeon's *Blue's Clues*, Mattel, and state health departments throughout the country. As founder and director of Moving & Learning (www .movingandlearning.com), Rae has been spreading the "movement message" since 1980.

Rae served on the original task force of the National Association for Sport and Physical Education that created *Active Start: A Statement of Physical Activity Guidelines for Children Birth to Age 5*. She is the author of eighteen books, including the three-book Moving & Learning series; *Physical Education for Young Children: Movement ABCs for the Little Ones*; *A Running Start: How Play, Physical Activity, and Free Time Create a Successful Child*, written for the parents of children ages birth to five; and the award-winning *Great Games for Young Children: Over 100 Games to Develop Self-Confidence, Problem-Solving Skills, and Cooperation* and *Jump into Literacy: Active Learning for Preschool Children*.

Additionally, Rae is cofounder of BAM! Radio Network (www.bamradionetwork .com), where she hosts the Internet radio programs *Teacher's Aid* and *Body, Mind, and Child*, and cohosts *NAEYC Radio*, interviewing experts in the fields of education, child development, play research, the neurosciences, and more.